Integrating Health
Impact Assessment
with the Policy Process

Integrating Health Impact Assessment with the Policy Process

Lessons and experiences from around the world

Edited by

Monica O'Mullane

Lecturer
Department of Public Health,
Faculty of Health Care and Social Work
(Fakulta Zdravotníctva a Sociálnej Práce)
Trnava University (Trnavská Univerzita), Trnava, Slovakia

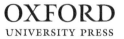

OXFORD
UNIVERSITY PRESS

OXFORD
UNIVERSITY PRESS

Great Clarendon Street, Oxford, OX2 6DP,
United Kingdom

Oxford University Press is a department of the University of Oxford.
It furthers the University's objective of excellence in research, scholarship,
and education by publishing worldwide. Oxford is a registered trade mark of
Oxford University Press in the UK and in certain other countries

First Edition published in 2013

Impression: 1

British Library Cataloguing in Publication Data
Data available

ISBN 978-0-19-963996-0

Printed and bound in Great Britain by
CPI Group (UK) Ltd, Croydon, CR0 4YY

Oxford University Press makes no representation, express or implied, that
the drug dosages in this book are correct. Readers must therefore always check
the product information and clinical procedures with the most up-to-date
published product information and data sheets provided by the manufacturers
and the most recent codes of conduct and safety regulations. The authors and
the publishers do not accept responsibility or legal liability for any errors in the
text or for the misuse or misapplication of material in this work. Except where
otherwise stated, drug dosages and recommendations are for the non-pregnant
adult who is not breast-feeding.

Foreword

Ildefonso Hernández-Aguado

The public health community has long been pursuing and advocating the adoption of healthy public policies as the best means to improve population health. However, changing public policies is always a difficult task, regardless of how knowledge-based the proposals are. The public health field has tried several strategies to promote healthy public policies with varying results. The very weaknesses of public health, its overstated devotion to health services, and the peculiar nature of the policy-making processes hinder the achievement of this key public health goal. In this context, health impact assessment (HIA) emerges as a more than promising tool to change practices and policies in wide sectors and to make them health sensitive. For HIA to achieve its full potential, we need pragmatic and balanced integration during the formulation of public policies. This book contains a broad range of practical knowledge and experiences, providing useful guidance to facilitate the incorporation of HIA in the decision-making process. The book's global perspective allows health advocates to encourage HIA application by showing how practices and experiences are implemented elsewhere and how public health laws have integrated HIA as a measure to maximize health outcomes when designing public policies. On the other hand, the relevant current studies described in the book boost new research that will enhance HIA development. Future research should improve the methodological tools, demonstrate the health gains and co-benefits on non-health policies which take health into account, and provide strategies to bridge the equity gap through HIA applications. There are now promising opportunities for HIA as the knowledge on social determinants of health is increasing and health and wellbeing is becoming a nuclear issue in modern societies. The need to make efficient policy choices by searching for the benefits in different domains, including health, will foster HIA implementation. This book is a unique resource in this endeavour.

Ildefonso Hernández-Aguado
Professor of Public Health, Miguel Hernández University, Spain
Former Director General of Public Health of the Spanish Government

Foreword

Debbie Abrahams

As a former HIA practitioner I am delighted to welcome this new book. It cannot be underestimated how valuable it is to have a contemporary collation of the experience of HIA practice across the world.

As a new politician I am convinced more than ever of the importance of HIA in policy decision-making and the implementation of policies based on evidence. Too often poor policy is implemented without any consideration during its development of the potential impacts it will have on the health and wellbeing of the population it is inflicted upon.

There are still many challenges for HIA: its relationship with other impact assessments, its use at national government level, the robustness and range of the methods and tools that are used, the vital importance of assessing impacts on inequalities (since the WHO Commission for Social Determinants 2008 report, it is unfortunate that a chapter on health equity impact assessment could not be included in this book's edition), governance arrangements, and HIA standards and quality.

We also need to ensure that development and learning in HIA are shared across the world. I look forward to future editions that will have chapters from contributors in China and South America, and more contributions from African countries.

Finally, although there are significant challenges for HIA, I believe there are also opportunities. There are legislative commitments in the USA, Europe, and a number of Asian countries that provide a valuable driver for HIA. Coupled with the personal commitment of HIA 'champions', these are the components for building and sustaining HIA, health in all policies, and a healthier world.

Debbie Abrahams FFPH
Member of Parliament for Oldham East and Saddleworth and
Parliamentary Private Secretary to Rt Hon Andy Burnham,
Shadow Health Secretary and a member of the Shadow Health Team

Foreword

Amphon Jindawatthana

Since 2000, the new era of health system reform in Thailand has unfolded. The reform has gone beyond health sector restructuring, making a paradigm shift in health concepts, directions, scope, ownership, and power relations within Thai society. Subsequently, public health responsibility does not only belong to the government, but is in the hands of all Thai people. Public health responsibility has not been limited to medical professions and the Ministry of Public Health, but has embraced all sectors. This shared responsibility opens up an opportunity for all sectors to be involved in formulating healthy public policy. The power relations have gradually been shifted to support and ensure the rights of people to determine their healthy life.

Among several innovations of the health reform movement in Thailand, the development of HIA has been proven as one of the most influential and successful changes. It is designed as a social learning process for all Thai people and will carry on as such. HIA researchers, practitioners, and the lay community have worked together to ensure that HIA will not turn out to be an exclusive technical tool for limited experts. Institutionally, HIA is stipulated within the National Health Act and also in the Constitution. HIA in Thailand aims not only to change the health sector perspective, but also the policy process and, above all, power relations in the country.

Thailand is one of the countries in this book that shares its practical knowledge and experience on how to use HIA to inform healthy public policy. There are not many books which describe the relationship between HIA and the policy-making process. This book is unique and plays a major role in advocating HIA for policy professionals and decision-makers. Although many countries reveal challenges for HIA in times ahead, opportunities can be found, in every step we take, if we walk together as a global HIA community.

Dr Amphon Jindawatthana
Secretary-General of Thailand's National Health Commission
June 2012

Acknowledgements

First and foremost I am deeply grateful to the chapter authors who contributed to this edited volume. Their determination in advancing the public health agenda in their respective countries and continents is nothing short of inspirational. May this book spread their knowledge and wisdom. The book's writing team are most grateful to the International Team of Reviewers who took the time and interest to review our chapters. Their contribution has undoubtedly improved the quality of our work. All authors and reviewers involved in this book play vital roles in developing HIA with their expertise, experience, and, most of all, genuine passion. I'd like to acknowledge those who have advanced the field of HIA for more than 20 years with their pioneering questioning and tenacity, and who particularly inspired my own love for HIA: Martin Birley, John Kemm, and Alex Scott-Samuel. My particular thanks to Mary Mahoney, Patrick Harris, Sarah Simpson, and my parents for their invaluable comments and fresh perspective on my writing, and to Professor Gareth Williams for his helpful observations on the initial proposal. Personally, I would like to thank some people in my life for their unwavering support, namely, my family (Mum, Dad, and Stephanie), my partner, Peter Kramá, my friends and mentors (in particular, Emmanuelle Schön-Quinlivan, Aodh Quinlivan, Julie O'Donnell, and Karen O'Mullane), and my colleagues in Trnava University (Slovakia) and University College Cork (Ireland) for their encouragement long before and during this editorial début! On behalf of the writing team, I would also like to thank the staff at Oxford University Press for their encouragement and patience during the book process. No question ever seemed too small and for that I am so grateful! Particular thanks to Nic Wilson, Caroline Smith, and Jenny Wright.

May we all continue to treat our home on planet Earth, and one another, in the respectful and kind manner as is embodied in the spirit of this book.

Contents

Contributors

Gifty Amo-Danso, MSc
Research Scientist,
IOM Centre for Health Impact
Assessment,
Institute of Occupational Medicine,
Edinburgh and London, UK

Judith Ball, MA, PGDipPH
Senior Research Associate,
Quigley and Watts Ltd,
Wellington, New Zealand

Dr Marleen Bekker
Post-doctoral Researcher
Department of Health Services
Research
Maastricht University
Maastricht, The Netherlands

Ben Cave
Director, Ben Cave Associates Ltd,
Leeds, UK
and
Honorary Fellow, School of
Environmental Sciences,
University of Liverpool,
Liverpool, UK
and
Chair, Section Co-ordinating
Committee,
International Association for Impact
Assessment
Fargo, North Dakota, USA

Dr Edith Essie Clarke
Programme Manager,
Occupational and Environmental
Health,
Ghana Health Service,
Accra, Ghana

Dr Noëlle Cotter
Public Health Development Officer,
Institute of Public Health in Ireland,
Dublin, Ireland

Dr Margaret Douglas
Deputy Director of Public Health,
NHS Lothian
Edinburgh, UK
and
Chair, Scottish HIA Network,
Scotland, UK

Professor Rainer Fehr, Dr med, MPH, PhD
Directorate, NRW Centre for Health,
Bielefeld, Germany
and
Professor of Public Health,
University of Bielefeld,
Bielefeld, Germany

Professor Thomas B Fischer, PhD, MIEMA
Head of Department for Geography
and Planning,
School of Environmental Sciences,
University of Liverpool,
Liverpool, UK

Gabriel Guliš
Associate Professor, Unit for Health
Promotion Research,
University of Southern Denmark
Esbjerg, Denmark

Dr Elizabeth Harris
Senior Research Fellow,
Centre for Health Equity Training,
Research and Evaluation,
Part of the Centre for Primary
Health Care and Equity,
University of New South Wales,
Sydney, Australia

Patrick Harris
Research Fellow,
Centre for Health Equity Training,
Research and Evaluation,
UNSW Research Centre for Primary
Health Care and Equity,
University of New South Wales,
Sydney, Australia

Ben Harris-Roxas
Conjoint Lecturer,
Centre for Health Equity Training,
Research and Evaluation,
Part of the Centre for Primary
Health Care and Equity,
University of New South Wales,
Sydney, Australia
and
Co-Chair Health Section of the
International Association for Impact
Assessment
Fargo, North Dakota, USA

Claire Higgins, MA
Public Health Development Officer
(HIA),
Institute of Public Health in Ireland,
Belfast, UK

Dr Martin Higgins
Senior Public Health Researcher,
NHS Lothian,
Edinburgh, UK
and
Co-ordinator, Scottish HIA Network
Scotland, UK

Dr Maria Jansen
Program Leader of the Academic
Collaborative Centre for Public
Health,
School of Public Health and Primary
Care (CAPHRI),
Maastricht University and Public
Health Service South Limburg,
Maastricht, The Netherlands

Dr Urmila Jha-Thakur
Lecturer,
School of Environmental Sciences,
University of Liverpool,
Liverpool, UK

Associate Professor Lynn Kemp
Director,
Centre for Health Equity Training,
Research and Evaluation,
Part of the Centre for Primary
Health Care and Equity,
University of New South Wales,
Sydney, Australia

Dr Jana Kollárová
Health Promotion Manager,
Department of Health Promotion,
Regional Public Health Authority,
Košice, Slovakia

Dr Pawan Labhasetwar
Scientist and Head,
Water Technology and Management
Division,
Council of Scientific and Industrial
Research,
National Environmental
Engineering Research Institute,
Nehru Marg,
Nagpur, India

Dr Piedad Martín-Olmedo
Senior Lecturer,
Escuela Andaluza de Salud Pública,
Granada, Spain

Owen Metcalfe, FFPH
Director,
Institute of Public Health in Ireland,
Dublin, Ireland

Dr Monica O'Mullane
Lecturer,
Department of Public Health,
Faculty of Health Care and Social
Work,
Trnava University (Trnavská
Univerzita),
Trnava, Slovakia

Dr Susie Palmer
HIIA Project, Project Manager
(Secondee from Glasgow City
Council, Health Policy Team),
Scottish Government Health
Directorates,
Scottish Government,
Glasgow, UK

Robert Quigley
Director,
Quigley and Watts Ltd,
Wellington, New Zealand

Arthi Rao
PhD Student and Research Assistant,
Center for Quality Growth and
Regional Development,
School of City and Regional
Planning,
Georgia Institute of Technology,
Atlanta, Georgia, USA

**Professor Mala Rao, MBBS, MSc,
FFPH, PhD, Hon FFSRH**
Professor of International Health,
University of East London,
London, UK
and
Honorary Adviser,
Administrative Staff College of India,
Hyderabad, India

Karen Roof, MSc
Graduate Instructor,
University of Colorado Denver
Denver, Colorado, USA
and
Principal,
EnviroHealth Consulting,
Denver, Colorado, USA

Dr Catherine L. Ross
Harry West Professor,
Director, Center for Quality
Growth and Regional Development
(CQGRD),
School of City and Regional
Planning,
Georgia Institute of Technology,
Atlanta, Georgia, USA

Associate Professor Louise Signal
Director,
HIA Research Unit,
University of Otago,
Wellington, New Zealand

Matthew Soeberg
Department of Public Health and
IAIA Health Section Member,
University of Otago,
Wellington, New Zealand

Dr Mieke Steenbakkers
Senior Policy Advisor Regional
Public Health Service South
Limburg,
Member of the Academic
Collaborative Centre for Public
Health,
School of Public Health and Primary
Care (CAPHRI),
Maastricht University and Regional
Public Health Service South
Limburg,
Maastricht, The Netherlands

Ilse Storm, MSc
Senior Researcher Health in All
Policies,
Centre for Public Health
Forecasting,
National Institute for Public Health
and the Environment,
Bilthoven, The Netherlands

Dr Decharut Sukkumnoed
Lecturer,
Faculty of Economics,
Kasetsart University,
Bangkok, Thailand

Francesca Viliani, MPH
Head of Public Health Consulting
Services and Community Health
Programs,
International SOS,
Copenhagen, Denmark
and
Co-Chair Health Section of the
International Association for Impact
Assessment,
Fargo, North Dakota, USA

**Dr Salim Vohra, MBChB, MSc, PhD,
FRSPH**
Director,
Institute of Occupational Medicine
Centre for Health Impact
Assessment,
Institute of Occupational Medicine,
Edinburgh and London, UK
and
Conjoint Lecturer,
Faculty of Medicine,
University of New South Wales,
Sydney, Australia
and
Honorary Fellow,
Faculty of Health,
Staffordshire University,
Stoke-on-Trent, UK

International team of reviewers

Dr Martin Birley
Consultant in Health Impact
Assessment,
London, UK

Dr Marcus Chilaka
Lecturer in Environmental Health,
School of Environment and Life
Sciences,
University of Salford Manchester,
Manchester, UK

Andrew L. Dannenberg, MD, MPH
Affiliate Professor,
University of Washington School of
Public Health,
Seattle, Washington, USA
and
Consultant,
Centers for Disease Control and
Prevention,
Atlanta, Georgia, USA

J.M. (Lea) den Broeder, MA MPH
National Institute for Public Health
and the Environment,
Bilthoven, The Netherlands

Dr Eva Elliott
Lecturer in Social Sciences,
and
Co-Director of the Wales Health
Impact Assessment Support Unit
(WHIASU),
Cardiff School of Social Sciences,
Cardiff University,
Cardiff, UK

Debra Fox, MRes, MCD
Department of Civic Design,
School of Environmental Sciences,
University of Liverpool,
Liverpool, UK

Dr Yoshihisa Fujino
Associate Professor,
Department of Preventive Medicine
and Community Health,
University of Occupational and
Environmental Health,
Kitakyushu, Japan

Patrick Harris
Research Fellow,
Centre for Health Equity Training,
Research and Evaluation,
University of New South Wales
Research Centre for Primary Health
Care and Equity,
University of New South Wales
Sydney, Australia

Fintan Hurley
Scientific Director,
Institute of Occupational Medicine,
Edinburgh, UK

Dr Mary Mahoney
HIA/HEIA Consultant and
Honorary Associate Professor,
Deakin University,
Melbourne, Australia

Dr Odile Mekel
Head of Section Innovation in Health,
Department Prevention and Innovation,
NRW Centre for Health,
Bielefeld, Germany

Anika Mendell
Research Officer,
National Collaborating Centre for Healthy Public Policy,
Institut National de Santé Publique du Québec,
Québec, Canada

Dr Lisa Pursell
Lecturer,
School of Health Sciences,
Health Promotion Research Centre,
National University of Ireland,
Galway, Ireland

Sarah Simpson
Conjoint Lecturer,
University of New South Wales (UNSW),
Sydney, New South Wales, Australia

Louise St-Pierre
Head of Projects,
National Collaborating Centre for Healthy Public Policy,
Institut National de Santé Publique du Québec,
Québec, Canada

Arthur Wendel, MD, MPH
Team Lead, Healthy Community Design Initiative,
CDR US Public Health Service,
Centers for Disease Control and Prevention,
Atlanta, Georgia, USA

Abbreviations

ADB	Asian Development Bank	EU	European Union
AHS	area health service	GIS	Geographic Information System
BRIA	business and regulatory impact assessment	HDMT	Healthy Development Measurement Tool
CBA	cost–benefit analysis	HEIA	health equity impact assessment
CHETRE	Centre for Health Equity Training, Research and Evaluation	HIA	health impact assessment
CHIA	child health impact assessment	HiAP	health in all policies
CPD	Community Planning and Development	HIIA	health inequalities impact assessment
CQGRD	Center for Quality Growth and Regional Development	HIP	Human Impact Partners
CVD	cardiovascular disease	HPP	healthy public policy
CVSFW	Service Framework for Cardiovascular Health and Wellbeing	HSC	health and social care
		HSE	Health Service Executive
		HSRI	Health Systems Research Institute
DBIS	Department for Business, Innovation and Skills	HSRO	Health System Reform Office
DH	Department of Health	HTA	health technology assessment
DHA	Denver Housing Authority	IA	impact assessment
DHB	district health board	IESIA	integrated environmental and social impact assessment
DoI	diffusion of innovation	IFC	International Finance Corporation
DPS	determinant policy screening	IIA	integrated impact assessment
EC	European Commission	IPH	Institute of Public Health in Ireland
EFHIA	equity-focused health impact assessment	LbD	l earning by doing
EHIA	environmental health impact assessment	LIGA.NRW	State Institute of Public Health
EIA	environmental impact assessment	LIHEAP	Low Income Home Energy Assistance Program
EMP	environmental management plan	MoEF	Ministry of Environment and Forests
EOI	expression of interest	NCD	non-communicable diseases
EPA	Environmental Protection Agency	NEPA	National Environmental Policy Act
EQIA	equality impact assessment	NGO	non-governmental organization
ER	environmental report	NHS	National Health Service

NI	Northern Ireland	QS	quick scan
NICE	National Institute for Health and Clinical Excellence	RFNP	Regional Land Use Plan
		RoI	Republic of Ireland
NIHPDP	National Institute on Health Promotion and Disease Prevention	SEA	strategic environmental assessment
		SEPA	Scottish Environmental Protection Agency
NRW	Nordrhein-Westfalen		
NSW	New South Wales	SFDPH	San Francisco Department of Public Health
OAU	Organisation of African Unity		
PEEM	Panel of Experts on Environmental Management	SHA	strategic health assessment
		SIA	social impact assessment
PHA	Public Health Agency	UDS	Urban Development Strategy
PHAC	Public Health Advisory Committee	UNECE	United Nations Economic Commission for Europe
PHS	Public Health Service	UNSW	University of New South Wales
PS	Performance Standards		

Chapter 1

Introduction

Monica O'Mullane

Nowadays, the view that our health is determined only by lifestyle and biological factors is neither plausible nor acceptable, given what we know about the wider determinants (influences) of health. Health is determined equally, if not more, by the environment (physical, social, cultural, and political) within which we all live (Jackson et al. 2011). The purpose of this book is to examine how health impact assessment (HIA) and the public policy processes in varying country contexts can be integrated. Since most countries across the world do not statutorily require HIA to be conducted, there are many unique and creative ways in which HIA can become more integrated with the public policy-making process. HIA needs to be integrated with the policy-making process in order to ensure health considerations are high on the policy and political agenda (Guliš et al. 2012). The aim of this book is to share these experiences and to examine how integration of HIA with the policy process can occur. The chapters are structured in such a way that each concludes with its own set of learning points, which are guides for reflection on the generic nature of the learning of each chapter, and can be transferred and applied across various cultural, country, and institutional contexts. It is the *principle* of the learning from each experience shared in this book, not solely the specific geopolitical context, which is integral to the book's overall message.

The Rio Political Declaration on Social Determinants of Health (WHO 2011) is a global political commitment that can provide a broadly global context for the subject of this book. The declaration calls for action to address the social determinants of health in order to reduce health inequalities and to improve health equity. The declaration calls for 'social and health equity through action on social determinants of health and well-being by a comprehensive inter-sectoral approach' (WHO 2011: 1). Following on from this, HIA was identified as a necessary instrument to enable inter-sectoral work and to improve public health by addressing the socio-economic determinants of health, so as to promote policies and practices that improve health equity and reduce health inequalities (WHO 2011: 5). HIA is increasingly cited and promoted as an appropriate and relevant approach that can inform public pol-icy-making processes by placing health considerations on the policy agendas. This book seeks to outline the worthiness of HIA and to equally outline the occasions in which it is not appropriate to conduct HIAs (Chapter 3).

Why this book?

The conception and hence creation of this book is a reflection of the growth of HIA practice and research globally, and its growing relationship with actors within the public policy-making system world-wide, from local through to international levels. This relationship continues to flourish, albeit not without growing pains; however, it progresses forward. The experiences shared within this volume reflect this fact. This book is the first of its kind to share global experi-ences of how HIA can be better integrated with policy processes in a variety of ways and means. It seeks to present the reader with relevant experiences in HIA research and practice that demonstrate the opportunities and challenges that exist in integrating HIA with policy processes. In the context of this book, inte-gration is a process, which may or may not be part of a state-driven institution-alization of HIA. The chapters in this book provide the conceptual foundation and analysis (Chapters 2, 3, and 18) and relevant global experiences (Chapters 4–17) that enable the reader to reflect on the selected range of experience.

The process of integration

Integration, indeed systematic integration, of HIA with the policy- and decision-making processes (Wismar et al. 2007) can often occur as part of the institutionalization of HIA in a country. This institutionalization could require policy support for the comprehensive (country-wide) embedding of HIA with policy-making procedures at local, regional, and national levels of government, which requires enabling factors such as policy support and polit-ical leadership, capacity-building, and resources for the institutionalization of HIA. However, in reality, it is often the case that a country does not have such a wide-ranging process of HIA institutionalization and instead a variety of activities are conducted to further the process of HIA integration with the policy-making system. This will be explored in this book.

The *Oxford Dictionary* (2012) defines integration as 'the action or process of integrating' or the intermixing of what was previously segregated. For the purpose of the integration of HIA with the policy-making processes, this book will demonstrate the variety of ways in which this integration can occur as a process that spans years in a variety of ways across countries, cultures, health systems, and institutions.

The plan of the book

The field of inquiry, namely the integration of HIA with public policy processes, will be the subject of Chapters 2 to 17. Chapter 2 discusses a range of conceptual roots of HIA, by describing first its multi-disciplinary nature, followed by an examination of the roots of HIA, namely public health and health promotion, with a specific focus on the determinants of health and health equity. Historical roots and policy drivers for HIA are also outlined. Impact assessment (IA) is described as another conceptual root for HIA, specifically its relationship with the public policy processes. Chapter 3 describes in greater detail the relationship between HIA and the policy-making processes. The chapter starts off by describing the healthy public policy (HPP) movement and health in all policies (HiAP) is also outlined. Instances when HIA is not the best option to take are given. HIA, as a tool for community engagement, is discussed in this chapter as well as its relationship to some key public policy-making theories, such as policy stages and policy analysis theories. These two chapters lay the conceptual foundation for the relevant experiences that are shared in Chapters 4 to 17.

Experts in the field of HIA who have worked not only in advancing HIA as a workable instrument, but have gone one step further in assessing the ways in which it may inform policy have contributed to this book. Chapter 4 illustrates the experience of the all-island Institute of Public Health Ireland in assessing the impact of HIA in policy-making in both Northern Ireland and in the Republic of Ireland, by analysing two HIAs conducted in each jurisdiction. One HIA was conducted on a health strategy (Service Framework for Cardiovascular Health and Wellbeing) and another on the Limerick urban regeneration project. Both cases are described and an analysis of how the HIA informed public policy is discussed. The chapter's learning illustrates the importance of the timing of HIA and the importance of the context that the HIA is taking place within. Chapter 5 also examines two jurisdictions' experiences in implementing HIA, albeit in geographically distanced locations within Europe: Denmark and Slovakia. The authors describe the differences and commonalities between the countries and the way in which HIA is being implemented by taking a wider public health system perspective and examining the process according to the Diffusion of Innovation (DoI) theory of Rogers (2003). Chapter 6 outlines a German experience with respect to spatial planning in the populated Ruhr area (Ruhrgebiet), a metropolitan region with approximately 5 million inhabitants located in the federal state of North Rhine-Westphalia (Nordrhein-Westfalen, NRW). Major cities in the Ruhr metropolitan area agreed to coordinate their spatial planning and develop a joint regional land utilization plan Ruhr (RFNP) as an innovative way forward. The State Institute of Public Health (LIGA.NRW; currently the State Centre for Health, LZG.NRW) provided a rapid HIA as a contribution to the spatial planning process. The consideration of the submitted health considerations by the planning authorities demonstrates the feasibility of HIAs being used to inform spatial plans. Chapter 7 presents us with the English experience on HIA and how it can have a role in shaping national government policy-making. This chapter shares experience on how HIA is embedded within the government impact assessment process and presents findings from an evaluation into how HIA is used by government departments (government ministries). The authors suggest that HIA must be aligned with allied approaches so that health impacts are routinely considered in national and international policies. Chapter 8 outlines the experience of HIA practice in the USA and highlights the major actors and institutions involved in HIA. Two case studies are described: an HIA of the Low Income Home Energy Assistance Programme (policy) and the Atlanta regeneration HIA (project). The chapter also identifies the connections between HIA and environmental impact assessment (EIA) in the USA. Chapter 9 presents us with the Australian experience, which provides an overview of the Australian workforce development programme intended to increase workforce capacity to undertake HIAs through a learning by doing (LbD) programme in order to address health equities. This was recommended by the New South Wales Health and Equity Statement *In All Fairness* (NSW Health 2004). The chapter describes the implementation of the programme, which trained state health officials to conduct HIAs. The authors conclude that LbD is an effective way of improving health system capacity in undertaking HIA. It is to be viewed, however, as one part of an overall reorienting of the health system for including HIA in mainstream population health practice. Chapter 10 provides us with the experience of HIA at local government level in New Zealand. The authors review the practice of HIA in the country since 2005 and critique the strengths and points for improvement of HIA practice in New Zealand. The chapter reiterates the importance of embedding HIA as part of institutional procedures in public health and local government, which involves, among other elements, leadership from key players and a strong commitment to addressing inequalities. Chapter 11 brings us the experience of Thailand and its story of HIA institutionalization since the beginning of the millennium. HIA in Thailand has been designed as a social learning process for promoting healthy public policy. In terms of legislation, HIA is safeguarded within the National Health Act (2007) and within the country's constitution. Future development of HIA in the country will focus on co-ownership for HIA so as to advance HIA as a societal learning process.

Chapter 12 outlines and describes how HIA can progress as a programmatic approach for HiAP in The Netherlands. The authors examine two studies that investigated the use and feasibility of HIA in The Netherlands and reassess the development of HiAP in the country. They conclude with recommendations of how HIA can be more succinctly aligned with procedures at local munici-pality level, by developing a more cohesive strategy that also facilitates middle-manager engagement. Chapter 13 describes HIA in India. The chapter explores the way in which health considerations are incorporated in Indian planning through impact assessments, mainly HIA and EIA. The authors appraise pub-lished examples of HIA reports and guidance, along with the Ministry of Environment and Forests' (MoEF) guidance for EIA. The authors subsequently examine the findings of a survey that sought to investigate the effectiveness of EIA in India and how EIA considers health and present recommendations for future incorporation of health considerations in impact assessment in India. Chapter 14 delves into the history of HIA in Africa, which reaches back several decades. HIA has not been conducted in a systematic way in Africa despite evidence of projects that impact negatively on health. This situation is chang-ing as government ministries and authorities across the continent are increas-ingly more aware of the need for inter-sectoral collaboration for planning for sustainable development. HIA was named as one of the key joint priorities at the first joint inter-ministerial conference on health and environment in Africa in Libreville (Gabon) in 2008. Chapter 15 describes the Spanish experi-ence of implementing and institutionalizing HIA. The chapter describes the incorporation of HIA into Spanish public health laws and examines the find-ings of a survey that elicited opinions from key informants on the challenges and opportunities associated with the process of HIA in the country. The author notes that although HIA is included in legislation, past experience warns against burdensome bureaucratization when implementing HIA, rec-ommending multi-disciplinary inter-sectoral collaboration at all levels. Chapter 16 outlines the challenges associated with integrating HIA with other IAs such as strategic environmental assessment (SEA) and equality impact assessment (EQIA) in Scotland. The chapter presents research into the consid-eration of health in SEAs and a pilot project regarding a new form of integrated impact assessment (IIA). The authors discuss the integration of health into other assessment frameworks to achieve better joined-up public policy formu-lation and improved public health. Chapter 17 examines the level of adoption of HIA recommendations for the South Lincoln Housing Master Plan in Denver, Colorado, USA. The author found that the HIA directly informed the planning process and policies as well as having an indirect impact and out-comes. The evaluation of this HIA suggests that HIA can play an important role in urban planning, as also highlighted in Chapter 6. Finally, Chapter 18 examines the lessons and experiences learned and shared throughout the book by analysing the patterns and commonalities amongst the various country and continental experiences. Discussion is structured between what is relevant and appropriate learning and reflection for practitioners and policy-makers, and for educators, researchers, and students.

This book's intended audience

This book has been written for a wide audience. It will be of use and interest to individuals working across all policy sectors in government ministries, departments, municipalities, and authorities. The book will certainly be of use and interest not only to professionals and practitioners working in public health, but equally for those working in adjacent disciplines and professions, such as the environmental sciences, spatial planning, and the political and social sciences. Non-governmental organizations (NGOs) and community advocacy groups will be interested in the lessons shared in this book. Students, educators, and academics will find this book helpful and insightful in their study, research, and teaching of HIA as a policy-support approach.

'Clean minds and dirty hands'

The approach taken for the book is based on the suggestion by the late Professor Geoffrey Rose (as also suggested by the *Journal of Epidemiology and Community Health*): to think, write, and present with both 'clean minds and dirty hands'. For the purpose of this book, this entails that the book is informed by a conceptual underpinning and by empirical observations and research, and practice. Chapters 2 and 3 provide background information on the relevant literature for HIA in terms of its conceptual foundations and its relationship with public policy. Global experiences are shared in Chapters 4 to 17, with Chapter 18 concluding on the lessons learned and the steps forward that can inform a post-Gothenburg international HIA consensus (Vohra et al. 2010).

Bibliography

Guliš, G., Soeberg, M., Martuzzi, M., and Nowacki, J. (2012) *Strengthening the Implementation of Health Impact Assessment in Latvia*. Copenhagen: WHO Regional Office for Europe.

Jackson, R., Bear, D., Bhatia, R., Cantor, S.B., Cave, B., Diez Roux, A.V., Dora, C., Fielding, J.E., Zivin, J.S.G., Levy, J.I., Quint, J.I., Raja, S., Schulz, A.J., and Wernham, A.A. (2011) *Improving Health in the United States: The role of health impact assessment*. Washington DC, USA: Committee on Health Impact Assessment. Board on

Environmental Studies and Toxicology, Division on Earth and Life Studies, National Research Council of the National Academies.

NSW Health (2004) *NSW Health and Equity Statement: In all fairness.* Sydney: NSW Department of Health.

Oxford Dictionary (2012) Available at: <http://www.oxforddictionaries.com/definition/integration>. Accessed 2 August 2012.

Rogers, E.M. (2003) *Diffusion of Innovations*, 5th edition. New York: Free Press, A Division of Simon & Schuster, Inc.

Vohra, S., Cave, B., Viliani, F. Harris-Roxas,B., and Bhatia, R. (2010), New international consensus on health impact assessment. *The Lancet* 376: 1464.

Wismar, M., Blau, J., Ernst, K., and Figueras, J. (2007) *The Effectiveness of Health Impact Assessment: Scope and limitations of supporting decision-making in Europe.* Copenhagen: WHO, European Observatory on Health Systems and Policies.

World Health Organization (2011) *Rio Political Declaration on Social Determinants of Health.* World conference on Social Determinants of Health, Rio de Janeiro, Brazil, 21 October. Geneva: World Health Organization.

Chapter 2

Health impact assessment: the conceptual roots

Monica O'Mullane

This chapter outlines the conceptual roots that have enabled and informed the development of health impact assessment (HIA). The multi-disciplinary nature of HIA is described, as well as its public health and health promotion background. The historical and policy drivers for HIA are discussed. The relationship that impact assessment (IA) frameworks can have with the policy process is described. This chapter provides a necessary description of the conceptual roots of HIA, which is empirically expanded on in Chapters 4 to 17.

A realistic perspective of HIA: a multi-disciplinary and inter-sectoral approach

Understanding the conceptual roots of HIA is necessary when examining its relationship with public policy. Although it is beyond the scope of this chapter (and book) to describe all of the influences on the development of HIA globally, this section aims to present an overview.

The assumptions underpinning HIA can be wide-ranging, depending on one's ontological standpoint (Haigh et al. 2012). HIA, as we know it today, has been with us for at least three decades, although the concept that all public policies affect public health is not new (Krieger et al. 2003). The 1990s represented a turning point, with calls being made for greater action around the promotion of HIA and its usefulness in informing policy development. Scott-Samuel's paper (1996) is cited as one of these calls whereby HIA was identified as a tool that should be advanced for better informed and improved public policy. Scott-Samuel later called for HIA to be developed as a 'key influence on evidence-based health policy' (Scott-Samuel 1998: 705). The Gothenburg Consensus Paper (WHO 1999) forms a broadly suitable underpinning for HIA conceptualization. The Consensus Paper proposed four values of HIA, encompassing an ethical framework for it (Birley 2011), equity, democracy, sustainable development, and ethical use of evidence, which set a high standard to aspire towards. The adoption of a comprehensive approach to health and a respect for human rights are additional values for this ethical framework (Scott-Samuel 2001; Birley 2011). The extent to which these values inform actual practice is the concern of the HIA community today (Harris-Roxas et al. 2012) as their goal is to ensure that HIA is not only used by experts, academics, and actors in the policy process, but is an instrument for community participation in local decision-making procedures (Mittelmark 2001).

HIA seeks to assess the impact of policies, programmes, and projects on public health across an array of areas, and across the public and private sectors (Krieger et al. 2003). The use and application of HIA methods and approaches has expanded rapidly over the past two decades in countries in all parts of the world (Harris-Roxas et al. 2012) and it is promoted by institutions such as the Organisation of African Unity (OAU), the World Health Organization (WHO) and the World Bank. The features of HIA indicate it is a multi-disciplinary approach, drawing on many diverse fields of study, from epidemiology, statistics, public health, and environmental health, to the political and social sciences, community development, and spatial planning (Kemm and Parry 2004a). It focuses on the multi-faceted interplay between the wider determinants of health, involves a wide range of stakeholders, a short time schedule for the HIA process, and has report production as an accepted norm (Mindell et al. 2004) thus enabling an inter-sectoral approach to address public health needs and concerns (Kang et al. 2011). Inter-sectoral action, defined as the participation and cooperation of various actors, is an integral part of public health research and practice (Lasker and Weiss 2003). HIA has been designed to ensure inter-sectorality of working between the sectors most commonly involved in HIA, such as public health, spatial planning, and environmental health, and by a range of community organizations, actors in the policy process, and research institutes (Lehto and Ritsatakis 1999). With regard to community organizations and, broadly speaking, citizen participation in HIA, many practitioners and researchers concur that HIA remains incomplete without both effective and instrumental community participation (National Centre for Healthy Public Policy 2011). However, the extent to which HIA can enable genuine participation as well as improving the scientific contribution is a topic of debate (Parry and Wright 2003; Kemm 2005; Elliott and Williams 2008; Harris-Roxas et al. 2012) as well as in other assessment frameworks (O'Faircheallaigh 2010; Esteves et al. 2012).

The Gothenburg Consensus Paper, as formulated by HIA practitioners, proposed the most commonly cited definition of HIA:

'Health Impact Assessment is a combination of procedures, methods and tools by which a policy, programme or project may be judged as to its potential effects on the health of a population, and the distribution of those effects within the population' (WHO 1999: 4).

This definition was expanded by Quigley et al. (2006: 1) to include the action-orientation focus of HIA (Birley 2011), thereby promoting the core purpose of why we have HIA in the first place, with an additional sentence at the conclusion of the abovementioned definition:

'... HIA identifies appropriate actions to manage those effects.'

As an approach and instrument to better inform public policy of the foreseen and unforeseen consequences of projects, programmes, and policies, and the fact that a comprehensive and social model of health underpins HIA, a core goal of HIA is to address inequalities in health. Inequalities are a result of the negative or positive effects of the determinants of health on various population groups, within countries or across countries and regions. The research of Wilkinson and Marmot in particular in highlighting the impact of the material and social environment on public health, through public policy, has been seminal through the work of social determinants of health, as shown in Figure 2.1. HIA adopts such a social model of health as its basis, differing from environmental impact assessment (EIA), for instance, which views

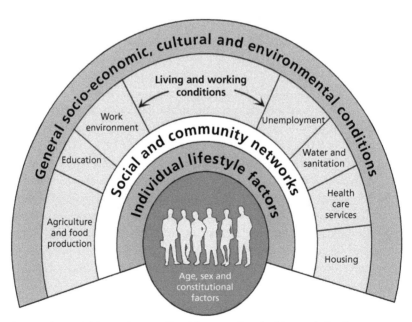

Fig. 2.1 The social determinants of health. Reproduced with permission from Dahlgren, G. and Whitehead, M. (1991) *Policies and Strategies to Promote Social Equity in Health*. Stockholm: Institute for Futures Studies.

health from a broadly biophysical perspective. The work of Wilkinson and Marmot emphasizes the dual importance of adequate material advantage, alongside a supportive social environment. That we require a well-rounded just and caring society for flourishing human beings is succinctly summarized in one sentence: 'As social beings, we need not only good material conditions but, from early childhood onwards, we need to feel valued and appreciated' (Wilkinson and Marmot 2003: 9). In 2008 the WHO Commission on Social Determinants of Health emphasized the relevance and necessity of HIA, especially in bridging the equity gap. The Rio Political Declaration (WHO 2011) on Social Determinants of Health identifies HIA as a necessary approach and instrument to address the social determinants of health and healthy equity of policies and practices.

Building the public health of the future: let's all play our part

The multi-disciplinary nature of HIA makes it a useable instrument for all professionals working in policy sectors such as transport, housing, economy, education, employment, and spatial planning linked to the physical environment, as much as it appeals to those working in community planning and development, public health, and health promotion. It provides a means of bringing together all willing partners in a particular policy process or project. Harris-Roxas and Harris (2011) argue that HIA is rooted within public health, and was conceived from three separate areas of activity (environmental health, the wider determinants of health, and health equity). It is important to approach HIA, theoretically and practically, with a multi-disciplinary mindset.

Much has been done at an international level to advance the holistic concept of health, since the WHO definition of health (WHO 1946) proclaimed that health is more than the absence of disease. Health for All by the Year 2000 was a programme for public health reform announced at the World Health Assembly in 1978 (WHO 1978). The subsequent *Health for All* strategy (WHO 1979) seminally highlighted that many of the factors affecting population health lay outside the healthcare sector, as was demonstrated by Marc Lalonde, as Minister of National Health and Welfare in Canada in 1974. HPP was an action area identified within the WHO Ottawa Charter on Health Promotion (WHO 1986). Since then, HIA has developed as an instrument that can advance the goals of healthy public policy (HPP; informing all public policy of health considerations), although both concepts can also operate independent of one another (Harris et al. 2012). The WHO-led Healthy Cities movement is also an effective model for building HPP (Ison 2009).

A significant redirection of the work of the WHO followed this announce-ment, resulting in an all-inclusive strategy for member states and the WHO itself (WHO 1981). The Health for All movement has been responsible for pro-moting (but has yet to achieve) equity and social justice as important societal goals (Lincoln and Nutbeam 2006). Subsequently, the Health for All in the 21st Century policy was launched in 1998 (WHO 1998). The member states of the WHO European Region thereafter formulated a new Health for All frame-work, *Health 21*, which included 21 health targets for the 21st century. This new policy aimed to achieve full health potential for all by endorsing three basic values: health as a fundamental right, equity in health and solidarity between countries, populations, sub-groups, and genders, and participation by and accountability of individuals and institutions involved in health development (Barton and Tsourou 2000). The strategy also called for the use of HIA in any programmes or policies that were likely to impact on public health (WHO 1998). Essentially, since the late 1970s there has been a growing awareness that much of the impact of decisions made in policy, programme, or project con-texts on public health exists outside the health system, and the work for health professionals lies in cooperation and participation with all partners engaged in and working outside the traditional healthcare sector. The WHO report of the Commission on Social Determinants of Health (WHO 2008) called for greater action from governments in addressing the broader determinants of health that lead to health inequities.

Work in promoting and addressing the impact of public policy on health has been strengthened, by moving the agenda forward. Health in all Policies (HiAP) is a 'complementary strategy with a high potential towards improving a population's health, with health determinants as the bridge between poli-cies and health outcomes' (Wismar et al. 2006: xviii). It builds on the triadic work of the WHO Health for All agenda, which calls for multi-sectoral action on health, on the concept of building healthy public policy, and on the whole government approach endorsed in the Bangkok Charter for Health Promotion in a Globalized World (Wismar et al. 2006). The HiAP movement focuses on strengthening the inter-sectoral action that is necessary for building HPP (Kickbusch et al. 2008).

HIA provides an appropriate mechanism to advance the public health agenda on local, national, and international levels, thus providing ample opportu-nities for informing health-sector and non-health-sector policy processes (Bambra et al. 2007; Harris et al. 2012). Although it is important that public health and health promotion professionals play their part and may lead the way, HIA is not an approach and instrument that can or should only be devel-oped and used by public health specialists; this is often the misconception.

It must also be pragmatic and relevant enough to be used (in terms of results and methods) and developed by all relevant professionals, such as policy makers, local authority officials, and community advocacy groups.

Health equity and health impacts

In 2008 the final report of the global Commission on Social Determinants of Health recommended that governments build capacity for health equity impact assessment (HEIA) among policy-makers and planners across all policy sectors (WHO 2008). This built on Sir Donald Acheson's 1998 recommendation for health inequalities impact assessment (Acheson 1998).

Underpinning the chapters in this book is the theme of health equity, as a core value of HIA (Gothenburg Consensus Paper) and both an explicit and implicit consideration of the role of HIA in addressing health inequalities and, potentially, health equity. In the light of the Commission's recommendation it is clear that considerable work will be required in the future on the links between HIA and specialist HEIA approaches, and the extent to which they have made a valuable contribution to the range of global activities linked to addressing health inequalities and inequities of policies.

This book demonstrates that there are multiple considerations that must be taken into account in respect to equity and inequalities depending on the stage of development of country, the intended purpose of HIA, or the overall capacity or capability issues in a country or region.

Chapter 9 explores in detail the New South Wales (NSW) HIA Project in Australia, which was initiated in response to the state level policy driver of considering health equity at policy level. The NSW Health and Equity Statement *In All Fairness* (NSW Health 2004) recommended the introduction of HIA and the development of processes for undertaking HIAs to ensure that proposed government initiatives would improve population health and minimize health inequalities. This chapter discusses this policy document, specifically the aspect that recommends HIA as an important organizational development strategy to increase the NSW health system's ability to address health equities. The capacities needed for conducting HIA and considering the health equity of the workforce required development in order to implement the policy's recommendation. The capacity building programme that ensued and the operation of equity-focused health impact assessment (EFHIA) is discussed and outlined further in Chapter 9.

Chapter 7 reminds readers of the importance of not losing sight of the end goal for HIA, i.e. that it can enable improved consideration of health and health equity impacts in policy-making processes. There is still much work ahead for

HIA practitioners and health officials to support and enable the development of the approach and monitoring of the extent to which its results are assimilated into improved public policy. The authors present the use of HIA and the consideration of health and wellbeing at national policy level in England. Their analysis indicates that across the government departments (ministries), the full range of social determinants was rarely considered and there was little focus on health equality and equity. The authors recommend that a monitoring process should be undertaken by the Department (Ministry) for Health, whereby instances when health impacts, determinants of health, and health inequalities and health equity are not being considered and should be are fed back to policy teams in order to enable improved consideration of health and equity in the policy-making process.

Chapter 4 focused on a specific application of HIA focused on equity, the HIA that was conducted on a Service Framework for Cardiovascular Health and Wellbeing (CVSFW) in Northern Ireland. The concept of a service framework, introduced by the Chief Medical Officer in 2007, was that it would reduce health inequities. HIA was identified as an approach that could be used to examine the potential impact of CVSFW implementation on health inequalities and inequities. During the process of the HIA, ideas were sought as to how to improve health outcomes through the CVSFW and avoid unforeseen effects on health equality and equity of service provision. The authors concluded that the HIA ensured the CVSFW would contribute to improving health equity considerations. Further discussion is provided in Chapter 4.

Chapter 5 compares the process of HIA implementation in Denmark and Slovakia, noting the influence of the WHO Europe and Slovak Biennial Collaborative Agreement workshop, which was established in cooperation with the Slovak Ministry of Health. The workshop focused in particular on the social determinants of health and equity within HIA and formulated the following recommendations for action: conduct pilot HIA case studies, further capacity-building on a regional level, and analyse the legislation from the point of view of mandatory environmental impact assessments with the inclusion of a health element. The potential outcome was an embedding of equity considerations in the HIA and EIA process in future. The capacity-building dimension was especially urgent given the impending enforcement of HIA legislation from January 2011. However, widespread HIA training with a focus on the social determinants and health equity throughout the regional authorities in Slovakia is yet to happen at the time of writing.

Chapter 10 outlines the central value placed on health equity in the development of HIA in New Zealand. Throughout all stages of the HIA process, the impact the proposal under scrutiny will have on communities is carefully considered. This chapter's experience illustrates that it is possible to conduct HIAs that address the social determinants of health and important values such as health equity, especially if it is an embedded principle from the start and matches the national agenda.

Finally, Chapter 14 considers the African experience. In this chapter, the authors suggest that the future of HIA on the African continent needs to include equity considerations so that vulnerable communities are not disproportionately affected. The authors call for improved understanding and visibility of equity in health within the African context.

Historical roots and policy drivers

Many countries have been influenced by the work of the WHO insofar as it has strongly advocated that HIA be placed on the agenda of respective member state countries. However, there has been much development worldwide on HIA practice since the Gothenburg Consensus Paper (1999) (Harris-Roxas et al. 2012), and many of the influences and policy drivers often originate from within country and regional boundaries. The proceeding chapters of this book (Chapters 4 to 17) illustrate this fact. As already mentioned, HIA has originated from within three broad areas of activity, namely, from within environmental health, the wider determinants of health, and health equity (Harris-Roxas and Harris 2011). Given the different emphases of these areas, there have been differing views about what role HIA should play (Harris-Roxas et al. 2012). Figure 2.2 illustrates this point, as well as highlighting some of the major milestones that have influenced the shape of HIA globally.

For many countries, the institutionalization of EIA has paved the path both for incorporating public health considerations into EIA and, further on from this, for the development of HIA. Although the institutionalization of environmental assessments across the globe is a noteworthy success, these assessments are often lacking the due consideration of human health impacts (Bhatia and Wernham 2008) that HIA brings to the table, so to speak.

For the African continent, almost at the same time as the Gothenburg meeting (1999), another meeting convened in Arusha, Tanzania (WHO 2001) to discuss the future ways of strengthening capacity in conducting HIA in African countries. It was decided that HIA practice would be progressed within the existing structures of environmental regulations (Chapter 14). In 2008 in Libreville (Gabon), the first Inter-ministerial Conference on Health and Environment in Africa was held. The goal of this conference was to attain commitment from African governments for reducing environmental threats to health; HIA is named as one of the 10 priorities of the Libreville Declaration (WHO 2001).

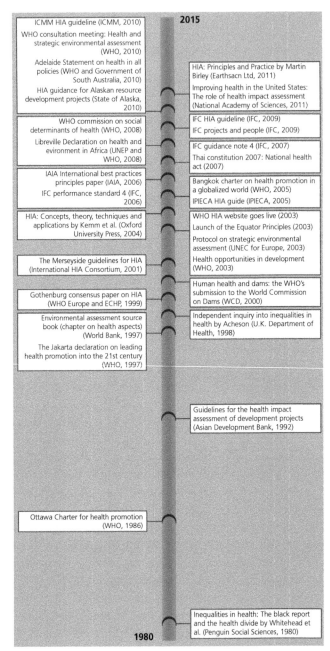

Fig. 2.2 Historical landmarks for HIA. Reproduced with permission from Ben Harris-Roxas et al., Health Impact Assessment: The State of the Art, Impact Assessment and Project Appraisal, Volume 30, Issue 1, pp.43–52, Taylor & Francis Ltd, copyright © 2012, <http://www.tandfonline.com>.

Impact assessment frameworks

When used in a policy context, Parsons (1995) argues that IA can be a useful policy-aiding instrument that can enable the analysis of possible positive and negative impacts that a policy decision may contain. Elliott and Williams (2008: 3) point to IA as a 'general approach to generating evidence for public policy' when it first evolved through the National Environmental Policy Act (NEPA) and EIA in the USA. Although IAs are traditionally used in a development project rather than in a policy context, from a policy scientific stand-point, they can be viewed and used as rational techniques informing the policy development process, and in producing evidence for public policy (Elliott and Williams 2008). Strategic environmental assessment (SEA), sustainability assessment (Bond et al. 2012), policy assessment (Adelle and Weiland 2012), policy IA, and some forms of integrated impact assessment (IIA) consist of some of the forms of IA that have traditionally focused on the impacts of policy and seek to influence policy. SEA and EIA can provide guidance through their experience for HIA institutionalization, in terms of both the experience of EIA and SEA in particular and incorporating the environment with health impacts (Dora 2004), as was demonstrated in the United Nations Economic Commission for Europe (UNECE) Protocol on Strategic Environmental Assessment to the Convention on Environmental Impact Assessment in a Transboundary Context (UNECE 2003).

In the consideration of the impacts on health of policies, HIA, and the policy-focused HIA (referred to sometimes as policy HIA) (Quigley et al. 2006), is an approach and term sometimes used to describe activities that examine the impact only of policies on public health (Mahoney, 2009). A suggestion by Joffe (2008) to rename what we know as the policy-specific or -focused aspect of HIA and policy HIA, to be called 'strategic health assessment' (SHA), is an apt recommendation that aligns separate policy-focused HIAs from those performed at project level, since currently the term 'HIA' refers to all types and levels of HIA. However, the SHA term is not in regular use (Mahoney, 2009) and the separation of upstream-level and downstream-level HIAs may be a disruptive move for this field of inquiry.

Rossi and Freeman (1993) broadly define IA as a framework of investigation within which the intended and unintended effects of policy can be estimated. They also acknowledge that definitive measurement of such policy consequences cannot be made with absolute certainty. However, it is not the aim of an IA to provide such a guarantee. Its central purpose is to evaluate the possible consequences of policy decisions, depending on the form of IA that is used, in order to better inform policy-makers of all options (Rossi and

Freeman 1993; Deelstra et al. 2003). An important point to note is that IAs are not envisaged as substitutes within the policy-making process, but are mechanisms to provide support for those formulating policy. The universal goal of all IAs, whether their primary focus be environmental, health, sustainability, social, poverty, equality, or regulatory, is to bring about a more ecologically and economically sustainable environment and equitable society developed through clear and accountable decision-making (Vanclay 2003).

Unlike other policy-aiding instruments, such as economic appraisal techniques, IA aims to facilitate a more participative decision-making process (Parsons 1995). It was originally envisaged within the context of EIA that it would 'become a valuable instrument for improving the political process', would engage relevant community stakeholders on an equal footing with elected policy makers and administration staff, and would enhance democratic wellbeing (O'Riordan 1976: 215). Indeed, in many instances it is striking how the courts, who must deal with challenges by environmental groups or individuals, 'have embraced the importance of EIA not simply as a technocratic aid to better decisions, but as a participative and democratic means of involving the public in decisions on projects' (Tromans and Fuller 2003: preface). It must be noted, however, that the participatory nature of IA, as learnt from EIA and social impact assessment (SIA) processes, in North America in particular, is quite complex and difficult to guarantee (Gregory et al. 2001; Ritsatakis 2004). When the NEPA of 1969 was enacted in 1970 after being passed by the Federal government, this marked the birth of EIA in the USA via the legislative route (US Congress 1970). It also marked the birth of an IA methodological family, from which subsequent forms of IAs would develop. Since then, many countries world-wide have legislatively institutionalized EIA, risk assessment, SIA, SEA, and other forms of IA. EIA originated as an action-forcing mechanism that was to coerce planners and decision-makers to incorporate the foreseen and unforeseen consequences of a project, programme, or policy into their final action plan (Caldwell 1982). Although the evolution of HIA differs markedly from that of EIA (Harris-Roxas et al. 2012), and has more in common with SEA in terms of its connection with policy processes, its relationship to other IAs is undeniable.

Health is considered in environmental assessments, but it is often considered within the biophysical health determinants as opposed to the broader concept of social determinants (Quigley et al. 2006) because these can be quantified and the potential significance of impact determined. Environmental health impact assessment (EHIA) exists essentially in order to incorporate HIA into or with EIA, in order to marry the two related concepts (Birley 2011), offering 'unique opportunities for the protection and promotion of human health' (Fehr 1999: 618).

There has been an ongoing debate in relation to integrating the foci of IAs into one IIA approach. Although the concentration into one IA is deemed practical for planners and policy-makers (Milner et al. 2005), no single declaration of what is best for all circumstances has been proclaimed. Instead, individual countries are encouraged to allow that 'local conditions (will) dictate a specific balance between integration and maintaining a separate profile for health in the overall impact assessment picture' (United Nations 2003: 116). The experience of Douglas et al. of an integrated assessment process provides more insight into this issue (see Chapter 17) and of the location of health in IA (Chapter 13).

Impact assessment within the public policy process

The study of HIA solely within the public and environmental health disciplines has expanded to incorporate the theoretical knowledge and experience that could be provided by the political sciences (Putters 1996; Kemm 2001; Banken 2001; Bekker et al. 2004; Wismar et al. 2007; O'Mullane and Quinlivan 2012). In fact, much earlier Milio, an advocate of the HPP approach, called for a new generation of policy studies that would be applicable for those developing HPP, within and outside government policy-making processes (Milio 1987). IAs are viewed as policy-aiding instruments, which are generally categorized under the umbrella of 'rational decision making' or 'rational techniques' (Putters 1996). However, these policy-aiding mechanisms can be used successfully, albeit differently, within other decision-making policy models (Bekker et al. 2004; Morgan 2008). No matter how rationally or logically policy-makers intend to operate, their institutional setting and context will influence the policy outcome. Instead of bowing to this pluralistic compliance, IA and all assessment techniques must adapt and become institutionalized appropriately into the policy-making arena, whilst accounting for pluralistic policy-making processes. A major issue that has arisen with the growth of IAs and the assessment framework is that when applied in project approval contexts, they may be burdens, or perceived as such, on the decision-making process. In this context the findings of an IA and of all assessment techniques need to be acknowledged and mitigated against in the approvals and implementation stage, with reduced burden on those within the policy process. It has been noted by those involved in IA and assessment techniques (Bond and Pope 2012) that this is a useful approach that continues to expand in bringing scientific evidence to the policy-makers' attention, and in ensuring that the local community affected by development projects is heard. Chapter 3 explores further the role of political sciences with HIA.

Concluding remarks: a necessarily multi-disciplinary approach

Although the idea that public policies affect health is not new, the systematic approach of HIA is novel. The success and acceptance of HIA by planners, policy-makers, practitioners, and community advocates lies in the use of its evidence in informing policy; this is its ultimate 'litmus test'. The HIA process must be central to or aligned with the policy-making process in order for health considerations to be duly acknowledged and accepted, when appropriate (Kemm et al. 2011; Guliš et al. 2012).

The conceptual roots of HIA, as we understand it today, originate from the HPP agenda and policy appraisal, from assessment frameworks (Kemm and Parry 2004a), and from the political sciences as a workable policy-aiding instrument (Lock et al. 2003; Milner et al. 2003). Although rooted in public health, the multi-disciplinary nature of HIA (Fabrizio and Paolo 2011) makes it an appropriate instrument as an inter-sectoral policy-aiding approach (Bekker et al. 2004).

This books aims to describe how HIA can inform policy development in various levels of government, in various settings and countries across the globe. The conceptual roots as outlined in this chapter are integral to the understanding and conceptualization of HIA as it operates globally, even allowing for unique national contexts. The following chapter explores HIA with a particular attention to the policy-oriented approach.

Acknowledgements

The author would like to acknowledge the invaluable input of Mary Mahoney and Sarah Simpson to this chapter.

Bibliography

Acheson, D. (1998) *Inequalities in Health: Report of an Independent Inquiry.* London: HMSO.

Adelle, C. and Weiland, S. (2012) Policy assessment and the state of the art. *Impact Assessment and Project Appraisal* 30 (1): 25–33.

Bambra, C., Fox, D., and Scott-Samuel, A. (2007) Towards a politics of health, in Douglas, J., Earle, S., Handsley, S., Lloyd, C., and Spurr, S.(eds), *A Reader in Promoting Public Health. Challenge and Controversy,* pp. 48–54. London: Sage and Open University.

Banken, R. (2001) *Strategies for Institutionalising HIA.* Brussels: European Centre for Health Policy.

Barton, H. and Tsourou, C. (2000) *Healthy Urban Planning*. London: Spon/Copenhagen: WHO.

Bekker, M., Putters, K., and van der Grinten, T. (2004) Exploring the relation between evidence and decision-making—a political administrative approach to health impact assessment. *Environmental Impact Assessment Review* 24: 139–149.

Bhatia, R. and Wernham, A. (2008) Integrating human health into environmental impact assessment: an unrealized opportunity for environmental health and justice. *Environmental Health Perspectives* 116(8):1159–1175.

Birley (2011) *Health Impact Assessment: Principles and Practice*. London: Earthscan.

Bond, A. and Pope, J. (2012) The state of the art of impact assessment in 2012 (Editorial). *Impact Assessment and Project Appraisal* 30 (1): 1–4.

Bond, A., Morrison-Saunders, A., and Pope, J. (2012) Sustainability assessment: the state of the art. *Impact Assessment and Project Appraisal* 30 (1): 53–62.

Caldwell, L.K. (1982) *Science and the National Environmental Policy Act—Redirecting policy through procedural reform*. Tuscaloosa: University of Alabama Press.

Carley, M.J. (1980) *Rational Techniques in Policy Analysis*. London: Heinemann Educational Books.

Committee on Health Impact Assessment (2011) *Improving Health in the United States: The Role of Health Impact Assessment*. Washington, DC: National Academies Press.

CSDH (2008) *Closing the gap in a generation: health equity through action on the social determinants of health*. Final Report of the Commission on Social Determinants of Health. Geneva: WHO.

Dahlgren, G. and Whitehead, M. (1991) *Policies and Strategies to Promote Social Equity in Health*. Stockholm: Stockholm Institute of Future Studies.

Deelstra, Y., Nooteboom, S.G, Kohlmann, H.R., van den Berg, J., and Innanen, S. (2003) Using knowledge for decision making purposes in the context of large projects in The Netherlands. *Environmental Impact Assessment Review* 23: 517–541.

Dora, C. (2004) HIa in strategic environmental assessment and its application to policy in Europe, in Kemm, J., Parry, J., and Palmer, S. (eds), *Health Impact Assessment: Concepts, Theories, Techniques and Applications*. Oxford: Oxford University Press.

Elliott, E. and Williams, G. (2008) Developing public sociology through health impact assessment. *Sociology of Health & Illness* 30 (7): 1–16.

Esteves, A.M., Franks, D., and Vanclay, F. (2012) Social impact assessment: the state of the art. *Impact Assessment and Project Appraisal* 30 (10): 34–42.

Fabrizio, B. and Paolo, L. (2011) Health impact assessment: a multidisciplinary procedure to support decision making in public health. *Epidemiolgoia and Prevenzione* 35 (2): 73–76.

Fehr, R. (1999) Environmental health impact assessment: Evaluation of a 10 step model. *Epidemiology* 10 (5): 618–625.

Gregory, R., McDaniels, T., and Fields, D. (2001) Decision aiding, not dispute resolution: creating insights through structured environmental decision. *Journal of Policy Analysis and Management* 20 (3): 415–432.

Guliš, G., Soeberg, M., Martuzzi, M., and Nowacki, J. (2012) *Strengthening the Implementation of Health Impact Assessment in Latvia*. Copenhagen: WHO Regional Office for Europe.

Haigh, F., Harris, P., and Haigh, N. (2012) Health impact assessment research and practice: a place for paradigm positioning. *Environmental Impact Assessment Review* 33: 66–72.

Harris, P., Haigh, F., Sainsbury, P., and Wise, M. (2012) Influencing land use planning: making the most of opportunities to work upstream. *Australian and New Zealand Journal of Public Health* 36 (1): 5–7.

Harris-Roxas, B. and Harris, E. (2011) Differing forms, differing purposes: a typology of health impact assessment. *Environmental Impact Assessment Review* 31 (4): 396–403.

Harris-Roxas, B., Viliani, F., Harris, P., Bond, A., Cave, B., Divall, M., Furu, P., Soeberg, M., Wernham, A., and Winkler, M. (2012) Health impact assessment: the state of the art. *Impact Assessment and Project Appraisal* 30 (1): 1–11.

Ison, E. (2009) The introduction of health impact assessment in the WHO European Healthy Cities Network. *Health Promotion International* 24: 64–71.

Joffe, M. (2008) The need for strategic health assessment. *European Journal of Public Health* 18 (5): 436–440.

Kang, E., Park, H.J., and Kim, J.E. (2011) Health impact assessment as a strategy for intersectoral collaboration. *Journal of Preventive Medicine and Public Health* 44 (5): 201–209.

Kemm, J. (2001) Health impact assessment: a tool for healthy public policy. *Health Promotion International* 16 (1) : 79–85

Kemm, J. (2005) The future challenges for HIA. *Environmental Impact Assessment Review* 25: 799–807.

Kemm, J. and Parry, J. (2004a) What is Health Impact Assessment? Introduction and Overview, in Kemm, J., Parry, J., and Palmer, S. (eds), *Health Impact Assessment: Concepts, Theories, Techniques and Applications*. Oxford: Oxford University Press.

Kemm, J. and Parry, J. (2004b) The development of HIA, in Kemm, J., Parry, J., and Palmer, S. (eds), *Health Impact Assessment: Concepts, Theories, Techniques and Applications*. Oxford: Oxford University Press.

Kemm, J., den Broeder, L., Wismar, M., Fehr, R., Douglas, M., and Guliš, G. (2011) *How can HIA support Health in All Policies?* Draft document presented at the Poznan Meeting of Polish EU Presidency, 8 November 2011.

Kickbusch, I., McCann, W., and Sherbon, T. (2008) Adelaide revisited: from healthy public policy to Health in All Policies [Editorial]. *Health Promotion International* 23: 1–4.

Krieger, N., Northridge, M., Gruskin, S., Quinn, M., Kriebel, D., Davey-Smith, G., Bassett, M., Rehkopf, D.H., and Millar, C. (2003) Assessing health impact assessment: multidisciplinary and international perspectives. *Journal of Epidemiology and Community Health* 57: 659–662.

Lasker, R.D. and Weiss, E.S. (2003) Broadening participation in community problem solving: a multidisciplinary model to support collaborative practice and research. *Journal of Urban Health* 80 (1): 14–47.

Lehto, J. and Ritsatakis, A. (1999) Health impact assessment as a tool for inter-sectoral health policy. A discussion paper for a seminar on 'Health Impact Assessment: From Theory to Practice', 28–30 October, Gothenburg.

Lincoln, P. and Nutbeam, D. (2006) WHO and international initiatives, in Davies, M. and MacDowell, W. (eds), *Health Promotion Theory*. London: Open University Press.

Lock, K., Gabrijelcic-Blemkus, M., Martuzzi, M., Otorepec, P., Wallace, P., Dora, C., Robertson, A., and Zakotnic, J.M. (2003) Health impact assessment of agriculture and food policies: lessons learnt from the Republic of Slovenia. *Bulletin of the World Health Organization* 81 (6): 391–398.

Mahoney, M. (2009) *Imperatives for Policy Health Impact Assessment: perspectives, positions, power relations.* Unpublished PhD thesis, Deakin University.

Milio, N. (1981) *Promoting Health through Public Policy.* Philadelphia: FA Davis.

Milio, N. (1987) Making healthy public policy. Developing the science by learning the art: an ecological framework for policy studies. *Health Promotion International* 2 (3): 263–274.

Milio, N. (2001) Glossary: healthy public policy. *Journal of Epidemiology and Community Health* 55 (9): 622–623.

Milner, S.J., Bailey, C., and Deans, J. (2003) Fit for purpose health impact assessment: a realistic way forward. *Public Health* 117 (5): 295–300.

Mindell, J., Boaz, A., Joffe, M., Curtis, S., and Birley, M. (2004) Evidence-based public health policy and practice: enhancing the evidence-base for health impact assessment. *Journal of Epidemiology and Community Health* 58: 546–551.

Mittelmark, M. (2001) promoting social responsibility for health: health impact assessment and healthy public policy at the community level. *Health Promotion International* 16: 269–274.

Morgan, R. K. (2008) Institutionalising HIA: The New Zealand Experience. *Impact Assessment and Project Appraisal* 26 (1): 2–16.

National Centre for Healthy Public Policy (2011) *Citizen Participation in HIA: An Overview of the Principal Arguments Supporting it.* Fact sheet, November edition. Quebec: National Centre for Healthy Public Policy.

NSW Health (2004) *NSW Health and Equity Statement: In All Fairness.* Sydney: NSW Department of Health.

O'Faircheallaigh, C. (2010) Public participation and EIA: Purposes, implications and lessons for public policy. *EIA Review* 30: 19–27.

O'Mullane, M. and Quinlivan, A. (2012) Health impact assessment (HIA) in Ireland and the role of local government. *EIA Review* 32 (1): 181–186.

O'Riordan, T. and Hey, R. (eds) (1976) *Environmental Impact Assessment.* Farnborough: Saxon House.

Parry, J. and Wright, J. (2003) Community participation in health impact assessments: intuitively appealing but practically difficult. *Bulletin of the World Health Organization* 55: 219–220.

Parsons, W. (1995) *Public Policy: An Introduction to the Theory and Practice of Policy Analysis.* Cheltenham and Lyme: Edward Elgar.

Putters, K. (1996) *Health Impact Screening: Rational Models in their Administrative Context.* Rotterdam: Erasmus University.

Quigley, R., den Broeder, L., Furu, P., Bond, A., Cave, B., and Bos, R. (2006) *Health Impact Assessment International Best Practice Principles.* Special Publication Series No. 5. Fargo: IAIA.

Ritsatakis, A. (2004) Health impact assessment at the international policy-making level, in Kemm, J., Parry, J., and Palmer, S. (eds), *Health Impact Assessment: Concepts, Theories, Techniques and Applications.* Oxford: Oxford University Press.

Rossi, P.H. and Freeman, H.E. (1993) *Evaluation Research.* Thousand Oaks, CA: Sage Publications.

Scott-Samuel, A. (1996) Health impact assessment. *British Medical Journal* 313: 183–184.

Scott-Samuel, A. (1998) Health impact assessment—theory into practice. *Journal of Epidemiology and Community Health* 52: 704–705.

Tromans, S. and Fuller, K. (2003) *Environmental Impact Assessment: Law and Practice.* London and Edinburgh: Read Elsevier.

UNECE (2003) *UNECE Protocol on Strategic Environmental Assessment to the Convention on Environmental Impact Assessment in a Transboundary Context.* Kiev: United Nations Economic Commission for Europe.

United Nations (2003) *Water for People, Water for Life: A Joint Report by the Twenty Three UN Agencies Concerned with Freshwater.* The United Nations World Water Development Report. New York: Berghahn Books.

US Congress (1970) *National Environmental Policy Act, 42 U.S.C. §4321.* Washington, DC:US Congress.

Vanclay, F., (2003) *Social Impact Assessment: International Principles. Special Publication Series No. 2.* Fargo, ND: International Association for Impact Assessment.

Wilkinson, R. and Marmot, M. (2003) *Social Determinants of Health: The Solid Facts,* 2nd edition. Copenhagen: WHO Regional Office for Europe.

Wismar, M., Lahtinen, E., Ståhl, T., Ollila, E., and Leppo, K. (2006) Introduction, in Ståhl, T., Wismar, M., Ollila, E., Lahtinen, K., and Leppo, K. (eds), *Health in All Policies— Prospects and Potentials.* Brussels: Ministry of Social Affairs and Health, Finland and European Health Observatory on Health Systems and Policy.

Wismar, M., Blau, J., Ernst, K., and Figueras, J. (2007) *The Effectiveness of Health Impact Assessment: Scope and Limitations of Supporting Decision-Making in Europe.* Copenhagen: WHO Regional Office for Europe.

WHO (1946) *Constitution of the World Health Organization.* Geneva: WHO.

WHO (1978) *Declaration of Alma-Ata International Conference on Primary Health Care.* Alma-Ata: WHO.

WHO (1979) *Formulating Strategies for Health For All by the year 2000.* Geneva: WHO.

WHO (1981) *Global Strategy for Health for All by the Year 2000.* Geneva: WHO.

WHO (1986) *Ottawa Charter for Health Promotion.* 1st international conference on health promotion, Ottawa, 21 November 1986, WHO/HPR/HEP/95.1. Geneva: WHO.

WHO (1998) *Health for All in the Twenty-first Century.* EB/101/8. Geneva: WHO.

WHO (1999) *Health Impact Assessment: Main Concepts and Suggested Approach* (Gothenburg Consensus Paper). Brussels: WHO.

WHO (2001) *Report of a partnership meeting on the institutionalization of HIA capacity building in Africa.* Geneva: WHO.

WHO (2005) *The Health for All policy framework for the WHO European Region: 2005 update.* Regional Committee for Europe. 55th session. Geneva: WHO.

WHO (2005) *Bangkok Charter for Health Promotion in a Globalized World.* 6th Global Conference on Health Promotion, Bangkok, August 2005. Geneva: WHO.

WHO (2008) *Closing the Gap in a Generation: Health Equity through Action on the Social Determinants of Health.* Final Report of the Commission on Social Determinants of Health. Geneva: WHO.

WHO (2011) *Rio Political Declaration on Social Determinants of Health, World Conference on Social Determinants of Health.* Rio de Janeiro, 21 October. Geneva: WHO.

Chapter 3

Health impact assessment and the policy process

Monica O'Mullane

Introduction

The purpose of this chapter is to lay a conceptual foundation to issues related to the policy process and health impact assessment (HIA), which will be explored further in the proceeding chapters. A description of the location of HIA within the healthy public policy (HPP) paradigm and an exploration of the problematic of HIA in relation to politics and society will be provided. The instances when HIA is not the best option to take will be discussed. The chapter provides a review of policy approaches and will demonstrate HIA's relationship to the policy-oriented approach. The role that underlying values and norms play in both the policy process and within HIAs themselves will be discussed. An overview of the policy actors potentially involved in HIA will be outlined.

Background

One of the main purposes of HIA is that it should support policy development, as 'a structured decision support tool' (Bhatia and Corburn 2011: 2410) by ensuring that the intended and unintended health impacts of proposals are duly recognized during or prior to policy formation. HIA is concerned with the biomedical and social health of populations. It seeks to enable policy-makers to inform policy with an evidence base. The rise of the evidence-based policy agenda in recent years, as well as the concept of a knowledge society (Jasonoff 2004), has been cited as influential drivers for impact assessment (IA) (including HIA) development. These have also been drivers for evaluation of its effectiveness and debate around its utilization in policy-making processes (Cashmore et al. 2010). This will be discussed further in the section on policy approaches to HIA. HIA activities, as well as the collection of data, aim to involve all relevant partners in the policy process and to ensure that evidence, as derived from this process, is used in policy development. The HIA process is concerned with the means as well as the ends (Banken 2001). That is to say, the process of HIA, which involves the networking of the relevant stakeholders across the varying sectoral domains and the raising of health on the agenda of policy makers, is as important as the outcome HIA report (Mindell et al. 2001).

Nevertheless, this normative underpinning of HIA is often unrealized. This book, with appropriately chosen current experiences, seeks to address this issue and share the unique and creative ways for integrating HIA with the policy process. Putters (2005) argues that efforts should not be spent only on defining HIA, but rather on investigating the policy context and process that HIA is expected to influence, integrate, and advocate. This is the purpose of this book: to examine how integration of HIA with the policy process can occur. Putters' call for a change in focus and attention on HIA epitomizes the change in activity and research on HIA. Prior to 2005, much HIA activity and research was centred on proving itself: as a concept, theory, technique, and method, and as a pragmatic response to concerns about the social determinants of health and health inequalities (Harris-Roxas and Harris in press). Post-2005 has been a period of broadening the focus to include examining whether HIA is used or not in policy and to directly or indirectly inform policy discourses, as has been evidenced by numerous research studies (Elliott and Francis 2005; Davenport et al. 2006; Wismar et al. 2007; Bekker 2007; Dannenberg et al. 2008; Ahmad et al. 2008; Kemm et al. 2011; Harris-Roxas and Harris in press; Harris, personal communication; Mahoney (2009) thesis).

The chapters of this book present some of the ongoing HIA global activity in evaluating HIA (Chapter 10), building capacity to address health inequities in the health system (Chapter 9), informing spatial planning (Chapters 6, 8, and 17), and the use of HIA and the consideration of health and wellbeing in national policy-level IA processes (Chapter 7). HIA can improve the health impacts of the built environment (Wendel et al. 2008; Dannenberg et al. 2011), as illustrated by chapters 4, 6, 8, and 17. The development of HIA and its impact on policies and strategies is also explored (*ibid*). Integrating health into impact assessments (Chapters 13 and 16), examining HIA implementation by comparing two European countries' experiences (Chapter 5), and the promotion of the inter-linkages of health and environmental considerations for improved policy-making processes (Chapter 14) are also topics explored in this book. Chapter 11 reflects experience in institutionalizing HIA through the legislative route and promoting it as a social process. Chapter 15 explores the perspectives of researchers and public health practitioners in the practice of HIA and its impact on the decision-making process. Chapter 12 examines the embedding of HIA as an instrument for advancing health in all policies (HiAP).

According to Putters (2005), the policy process and the organizational culture unique to each institutional context require examination that should supersede all research pertaining to HIA. Others have argued that if the instrument is rendered as a misunderstood administrative burden and barrier to policy initiative then it will be cast aside by decision-makers in the policy process (Parry and Stevens 2001; Krieger et al. 2003; Kemm et al. unpublished). Although continued development of relevant, reliable, and workable methods for HIA is vital, there also needs to be continued dual recognition of aligning and integrating HIA with the policy processes. Efforts are required to ensure HIA is viewed as a positive process, seeking to improve positive outcomes and decrease negative outcomes from the policy process (WHO 2012). Although the debate regarding the understanding of the policy process and its relationship with HIA is still a relatively novel field of inquiry (Milner et al. 2003; Bekker 2007), it is increasingly viewed as an area requiring further research. In light of the voluntary status of HIA in most countries, in contrast to the statutory recognition of environmental impact assessment (EIA) and strategic environmental assessment (SEA), proactive research into the understanding of the policy process is even more urgently required if HIA is to have a chance at integrating its process and its derived evidence.

For the purpose of this chapter, the term 'decision-maker' relates to an individual or group of individuals (deemed the decision-maker) authorized by the state who are involved in decisions within the official state, intergovernmental, or supranational policy process. This group of individuals generally are in a position of power required to make and implement the decision. The term 'policy-maker' refers to individuals who develop policy proposals and are often involved in implementation. Decision-makers and policy-makers are often not synonymous but usually both groups operate within local, regional, and national tiers of governance.

HIA: informing HPP and advancing HiAP

Milio highlighted in the 1980s the important effect that public policy has on population health, and the necessity that exists to assess policies for their health impacts (Milio 1981). This concept was adopted within the Ottawa Charter for Health Promotion by the WHO (1986) as one of its five key action areas for health-enhancing public policy: HPP. As a policy instrument it is within HPP (St.Pierre 2007; Collins and Koplan 2009; Kemm et al. 2011) that HIA is located by predicting both expected and unexpected consequences of projects, programmes, and policies, and also by informing policy-makers of such consequences. In order to do so, building support for HIA within policy and institutional arenas is necessary, as well as integrating HIA into the policy-making process (Kemm et al. 2011). Adequately predicting and managing these possible effects, and informing the policy process of the identified effects of different policy options, are not synonymous concepts; they require at some times separate, and at all times appropriate, methods, approaches, and conscious strategic planning.

Combined, HIA as an approach (Wismar 2007) meets two generally accepted conditions for healthy public policy (Kemm 2001: 80):

1. The health consequences of different policy options have to be correctly predicted.
2. The policy process has to be influenced so that health consequences are considered.

Whether or not HIA can be or is a cornerstone to HPP has been the subject of debate (Metcalfe and Higgins 2009; Morgan 2009). Harris (forthcoming thesis) provides a novel analysis of the relationship between HIA and HPP, concluding that the two concepts are separate and can operate independently but are mutually supportive. HIA is an instrument that can enable the methodical inclusion of health in public policy, whilst HPP (and more recently HiAP) is broader in scope and concept, based on a wider sense of inter-sectoral collaboration. Additionally, and most importantly for policy-focused HIA research and practice, both HIA and HPP are influenced by that which they attempt to influence: public policy. In order to influence public policy, we need to understand its processes, underlying values, and approaches (Harris, forthcoming thesis) (the section on policy approaches and HIA explores this further). This will enable the process of integration of HIA with the policy process.

However, the success of HIA in evolving as an approach for ensuring healthy public policy is dependent on a number of recurring themes that HIA practitioners and researchers have advocated at previous international HIA conferences, such as political leadership is a vital ingredient in using HIA evidence in policy, local government structures for policy-making enables the use of HIA, managing stakeholder expectations of HIA is important, policy planning processes can be a gateway for HIA to achieve HPP and in advancing HiAP, and the decision makers in the policy process must be included in the HIA projects from the beginning.

When HIA is not the best option to take

There are times when it is not appropriate or relevant to conduct an HIA. HIA is not designed as a 'magic bullet' (Taylor and Blair-Stevens 2002: 4) or as the only option for informing policy development of health impacts. There are three main instances when HIA may not be the best option to take. Firstly, it may be more appropriate to conduct another assessment, for instance an environmental assessment (SEA), or to include health considerations as part of an IIA. Which assessment framework should be implemented is contingent on its aims and goal; what is to be expected of the assessment. Secondly, if a government ministry requires that a health economic appraisal is to be conducted of a policy proposal, for example for a national playground programme, it is probably more appropriate to initiate a cost–benefit analysis (CBA) rather than an HIA. Thirdly, if a stakeholder in the HIA process, for instance a decision-making local authority, is included in an HIA but has no power or has no intention to amend the proposed policy, then conducting an HIA may only cement any inter-agency tension and be a loss of time, energy, and work. Planning the type of HIA (desk-top, intermediate, comprehensive) also will take time and consideration, as sometimes it is more feasible and relevant for the policy process (both in terms of the evidence needed and the timing of decision-making within the policy process) that a desk-top HIA be conducted rather than a comprehensive HIA.

However, due accordance for each individual context needs to be noted. Whether or not to undertake an HIA, or which type of HIA to conduct, will always depend on context-specific factors, such as timing, data availability, and the willingness of key stakeholders to engage with the process. Indeed, it is sometimes necessary to balance the need for updated information 'with the realities of varying data quality' (Jackson et al. 2011: 10).

HIA and society: 'leave the science to the scientists'?

As mentioned in Chapter 2, there is a debate regarding the relationship between HIA and community participation. There is a perceived tension between the perspectives of HIA, it being viewed as a rational technique (objective) and as a social process (subjective). The two perspectives may sometimes be seen to be at odds with one another, since enabling public participation in HIA as well as the development of HIA as an instrument that presents scientific information may prove to be a difficulty (Parry and Wright 2003; Kemm and Parry 2004), especially for states seeking to institutionalize the approach. Given that one of the HIA values (suggested by the Gothenburg Consensus Paper) is democracy, which advocates that the power to rule be invested in the people, it is an important aspect to address. HIA involves the collection of knowledge in order to inform the policy process, and the role of public participation is inherent in both the political nature of the IA framework (Cashmore et al. 2010) and the political nature of the policy system.

Birley (2011: 132) rightly declares that 'HIA is based on an interpretative rather than positivist approach to science'. This not to say that the positivist aspects of HIA are null and void, as its underlying normative rationality denotes positivism. However, in examining HIA from a policy-informing and -analytic perspective, HIA comes more under the post-positivist umbrella, thus not 'leaving the science to the scientists' only. The tension between the perceived intractability between these two perspectives, objective knowledge versus subjective knowledge (which includes public participation), is mirrored in the historical tension within the policy sciences. Howlett et al. (2009: 21) put forth the 'meta-approaches to studying public policy', which include the positivist approach to policy analysis (a deductive and prescriptive approach to policy analysis focusing on linking quantifiable policy outcomes with policy determinants), the post-positivist approach (a counter-perspective to positivism, which rejects the notion of quantifying outcomes without due recognition of social context and the politics of the policy process), and post-structuralist (denies the presence of objective facts that are separate from subjective observations). These approaches are helpful in observing, understanding, and analysing policy-making and their respective elements can co-exist (Knoepfel et al. 2007; Howlett et al. 2009). However, it is important for both those seeking to influence the policy process and those working within the process to be mindful of these broad approaches to policy analysis. For full policy analysis, positivist and post-positivist approaches are necessary (Howlett et al. 2009). Equally, in relation to knowledge gathered within the context of an HIA, Elliott and Williams (2008: 4) highlight that bearing the assumption that knowledge gathered by positivist means and knowledge gathered via the lay community are two kinds of knowledge may lead to a misguided definition of what is 'legitimate evidence'. There is, however, no reason why these two forms of knowledge cannot complement one another. As those involved in HIAs can illustrate (for instance in Chapters 4, 10, and 17), lay knowledge and community participation can often lead to a more comprehensive description of the context for the HIA, thus leading to a better informed process and outcome report, and recommendations for policy.

The question is: can these two faces of HIA coexist without negating one another? HIA as a social process and mechanism for health reform is illustrated in Chapter 11 by the Thai experience, which demonstrates how HIA, as outlined originally in Thailand as a social process, can be well integrated into the institutional structures and as an identified instrument for public participation. Adjustments may be made in the future; however, the Thai experience does provide the HIA community with some hope as to how institutionalization with a focus on public participation can be done.

Policy approaches and HIA

This section will provide a brief overview of policy and politics definitions in order to guide the following discussion of policy approaches. The research conducted to date, which sought to link various policy approaches with public policy, will be discussed. Although much work has been done to date (Bekker et al. 2004; Putters 2005; Wismar et al. 2007; Kearns and Pursell 2011; Kemm et al. 2011) that examines the relationships between HIA and the policy process, it is necessary to examine to what extent practice illustrates the extent of an integration between HIA and policy-making, integration being a process. Whether current practice aligns itself with the norms, rationales, and practicalities of the policy-making arena will be discussed in Chapter 18.

Policy definition has attracted much speculation but little conformity. At the risk of attempting to define what Wildavsky (1979) considers the indefinable, key explanations of policy conceptualization will be illustrated. The essence of 'policy' is that it entails purposive action on the part of the policy-maker (Walt 1994) in dealing with a problem or issue of concern (Hogwood and Gunn 1984). Heclo (1972) describes the concept as courses of action rather than the particular decisions themselves; it is the process, not the outcome, which Heclo believes encompasses 'policy'. Public policy has been described as a 'choice' that governments take in deciding what action to choose, and alternatively what not to take (Dye 1976). Policy extends, however, beyond the concrete choices made on behalf of the policy-makers and decision-making actors in the process, all inter-related in a web of policy processes and capabilities to act on issues (Howlett et al. 2009). Since the work of Aristotle, and his assertion of the 'polis' being the highest form of human association, a search has continued for a negotiation of the tension between the public and private realms of human activity.

Politics is an activity associated with policy-making, which is one of the key determinants of policy outcome and impact. Summed up astutely by one of the founding fathers of the policy sciences, Harold Lasswell (1935) defines politics as the battle over 'who gets what, when, and how'. For some, politics is the study of power (Jordan and O'Riordan 2001). Power can be exercised in the form of violent coercion or, more subtly, through factors associated with social norms, values, and processes (Cashmore et al. 2010). It is important for HIA practitioners and those involved in HIAs to be aware of the role that politics, policies, and indeed political regimes play in the process and eventual use of HIA evidence. This is demonstrated in Chapter 5, with the comparison of HIA implementation in Slovakia and Denmark. The impact of public health policy systems on HIA development and implementation is discussed in this chapter. Indeed, Chapters 4 to 17 all highlight in varying ways the impact of policy systems on HIA development, implementation, and use of its evidence in policy-making.

Since HIA is operating in a political and policy climate when it seeks to integrate its evidence within the policy process, the goal must continue for HIA practitioners to present policy-makers with a variety of policy options which explicitly outline their respective trade-offs. Petticrew et al. (2004), concluding from a study which involved the querying of decision-makers about how research evidence influences public health policy making, called for unbiased and objective evidence as a primary request or need. This research relays important information for those involved in HIA practice, and for those who are destined to use evidence from HIA. The task of the HIA, its process and its concluding report, is to present evidence in an objective manner and to indicate to decision-makers what the explicit trade-offs and uncertainties for each policy options are within the various alternatives (Mindell et al. 2001). However, there is sometimes a blurring of the understanding of HIA's role: as an advocacy instrument, as a means to present impartial knowledge and evidence, or both (Kemm 2011).

Where influencing the policy process is concerned, HIA operates as a political activity and a course of action which requires connection within the political structures (Taylor and Blair-Stevens 2002). Indeed, IA frameworks are expected to, in the very least, generate greater attention in policy development on a specific issue (Cashmore et al. 2010). IAs (including HIA) have been labelled by Cashmore et al. (2010) as policy integration tools, and the degree of integration depends on context-specific factors, such as the policy actors involved and their underlying values and expectations, and the political and institutional system's constraints and opportunities. If HIA requires a connection with political structures, then it logically follows that a due understanding of how the political system and policy-making processes operate is required. As both practitioners involved in HIA and as professionals working within the policy process, an exploration of the policy models in the literature and those used in practice can assist in better understanding how HIA can integrate or align with policy processes. This can lead to greater awareness of the facilitators and barriers to integrating HIA with the policy process, thus enabling an amendment of actions and processes in accordance.

Much previous work has been done regarding HIA and the policy process, some of which will be outlined in this section. Bekker et al. (2004) examined the interaction of HIA and decision-making, concluding that by mapping the policy process HIA practitioners can optimize the use of HIA and produce an appropriate HIA. The authors examined rational, incremental, and mixed models of decision-making to examine the use of HIA evidence by decision-makers. Putters (2005) investigated three models of HIA that are connected to relevant policy-making models: that HIA can fit with a rational idea of policy-making, with a rounds (Echternach) model, and with a 'garbage can' model. These models are envisaged to optimize health interests in policy-making. HIA has been found to influence the policy process indirectly (Elliott and Francis 2005). Indeed it has been found that effects of policies are oftentimes not realized or experienced by the public for many years after a particular policy action (Scott-Samuel 2006). Wismar et al. (2007) evaluated HIA effectiveness in policy-making by looking at the degrees of effectiveness across various country cases.

Rationalism and incrementalism

The nature of decision-making processes are often contingent on the policy issue, the actors involved, the institutional and informational contexts, and pre-existing decision-making routines and ideas (Howlett et al. 2009). Such variables are present in some form or another in various decision situations, and the particularity of the circumstance will evoke certain decision-making approaches. There have traditionally been two approaches to decision-making: the rational model (which purports that a scientific gathering of information and screening of policy options can be performed) and the incremental model (which states that decision-making has less to do with technical gathering of data and more to do with bargaining and negotiation). The mixed-scanning model was developed as a response to the aforementioned polar-opposite models, seeking to merge elements of rationality and incrementalism (Etzioni 1967). Since the 1980s, there has been a growing awareness that the debate between rationalists and incrementalists has evolved into a recognition that a holistic understanding of the policy process (accounting for rational and incremental leanings) and the role that subsystems play in policy-making is important (Etzioni 1967). Gagnon et al. (2007) demonstrate the usefulness of taking a subsystem approach to policy-making in their study examining the formation of HPPs. In HIA research and practice, practitioners in the field need to be more conscious of the public policy decision-making climate and, as demonstrated by Bekker et al. (2004), can adequately inform the process when armed with knowledge of the approaches to decision-making. However, it must still be acknowledged that 'a rational assessment (IA) for an irrational context (policy-making arena) is often difficult' and can at times dilute the impact of the HIA in informing policies and programmes (O'Mullane and Quinlivan 2012: 186).

The policy stages approach and HIA

There has been a development of the rationality of the term 'policy' as being quite distinct from the passion and subjectivity associated with 'politics' (John 1998). This rational development has laid the foundation for the progression of the policy-analytic, or policy-oriented, approach (Ham and Hill 1993; Howlett et al. 2009). This approach, of simplifying the complexity of public policy-making into a number of distinctive components, originates in the work of Lasswell (1956; 1959). This stages approach makes policy more amenable for analysis (Ham and Hill 1993), although it has not been without criticism (Sabatier 1999; Lindblom and Woodhouse 1993).

It is important to note that policy making is a 'complexly inter-active process' and the policy cycle rarely takes the linear form as is theorized (Lindblom and Woodhouse 1993: 11). Stages can be interwoven and it is more useful to view policy-making as an iterative process including these stages than anything inherently rational. For the purpose, however, of examining how HIA can relate to the stages or elements of policy-making, the policy cycle approach provides essential insight and information.

As Figure 3.1 illustrates, there are five stages of the policy cycle. Howlett et al. (2009) provides an excellent analysis of these stages, which are overviewed briefly here. The agenda-setting stage refers to the issues or problems which are the focus of the policy actor's attention, those both inside and outside political structures, and how they are prioritized. Policy formulation is associated with

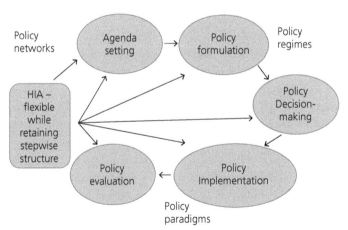

Fig. 3.1 HIA and policy-making. Reprinted from Harris, P., Sainsbury, P. and Kemp, L, HIA and Public Policy Internationally: Essential Elements for Sustaining HIA, Plenary Session 'How to make HIA stick' – Inaugural National Health Impact Assessment Meeting, April 3-4th, Washington DC, Copyright © 2012 with permission from the author.

producing options on what action to take (or not take) on a public issue. Policy decision-making is the stage within which the issues discussed and investigated throughout the previous stages are generated into policy options. These options will be decided on by the relevant decision-makers, usually generated in a formal or informal declaration of action to be taken. Policy implementation refers to acting on the decisions made previously. Policy evaluation, when combining 'elements of both the positivist and post-positivist perspectives' (Howlett et al. 2009: 179) can be regarded as a stage of policy learning. The benefit of taking the 'policy learning' approach to evaluation is to broaden the scope for assessing the policy, i.e. its impact on the policy sector, policy actors, and in informing future policy directions.

Harris (forthcoming thesis; personal communication), using the Howlett et al. framework, suggests the following as an analysis of the relationship between HIA and the policy-making process.

Each stage of the cycle influences and can be influenced by HIA. Agenda-setting sets the stage for what HIA could assess as public policy issues. HIA as a technical policy process fits best in policy formulation (remembering that even policy formulation is non-linear and may appear at different points in policy-making). Decision-making is nested within agenda-setting and formulation, and is ultimately what HIA aims to influence. HIA can also be used to influence policy implementation as part of the 'policy mix' of instruments used. HIA should also attempt to influence policy learning (social, conceptual, and technical learning, both inside and outside government) alongside or through policy evaluation.

Outside the cycle there are a number of further contextual influences, the policy subsystem, on policy-making made up of institutions, ideas, and actors. Essentially the policy subsystem includes policy networks (including interactions inside and outside government between government and social organizations), policy regimes (involves the impact of long-running policy development influenced by actors, institutions, and ideas), and policy paradigms (assumptions that may limit action by constraining the policy options available). The arena impacts on the policy cycle by constraining or enabling activity, including HIA, depending on the national or local context (Harris, forthcoming thesis).

The role of values in the policy process

It is important to account for the role which values play within the policy process, and within HIAs, when endeavouring to understand the processes of both. Indeed, Bekker (2007) highlights a key role that HIA plays to make the values of all the policy sectors involved more visible. The experience of Denmark and

Slovakia (Chapter 5) highlights the longer tradition of democracy in Denmark for smoother implementation of the values of HIA. The authors conclude that a social system which supports the values of HIA is an enabling factor for its implementation. Research conducted regarding HIA practice in Spain highlighted the challenge of integrating holistic public health values across all policy sectors, as the basis for HIA. Scottish experience in relation to integrating health into IAs (Chapter 16) brings to our attention the need to be mindful of the varying values underpinning IAs. The differences and commonalities between IAs may explain why some IAs are easier to integrate with one another than others. It is important that those working in HIAs and from within the policy process are mindful of the values underpinning the IA, sector, political system, and structures.

Easton (1953) notes how 'policy' is a network of decisions and activities, and the values of the decision-maker underscore the specific policy. Indeed, since the foundation for the policy sciences was constructed, there has been greater recognition of the role that values play in the processes of policy making (Weiss 1977; Gagnon et al. 2007) and this has been highlighted in policy-oriented research for HIA (Elliott and Francis 2005). Bekker et al. (2004) concluded that the values of decision-makers are an important factor, as well as maintaining constant communication with decision-makers. This point was reiterated in Bekker (2007) (overviewed in Chapter 12), who concluded that there can be a tension between the value-ridden policy process and an objective outline of health impacts. O'Faircheallaigh (2009) analysed the role of values in relation to decision-maker values of sustainability and their significant impact on the policy process. Cashmore et al. (2010) propound those actors' beliefs, both in the conduct of IAs and in the policy process where evidence is used or not, is an important consideration. Values and beliefs (for example, how is health viewed, and which is valued more, cost-effectiveness or an appropriate yet costly intervention?) are essential in how an IA is understood and used. This is an imperative aspect to be aware of for the integration of HIA with public policy, as was demonstrated in the use of HIA evidence in local policy in Northern Ireland and the Republic of Ireland (O'Mullane 2009).

Policy analysis: the art and craft (Wildavsky 1979)

As was stated already that it is vital for both those seeking to influence the policy process and those working within the process to be aware of the approaches to policy analysis: broadly, positivist and post-positivist. For full policy analysis, both approaches are needed to devise a deductive and interpretative perspective for policy analysis.

Policy analysis is a branch of study that seeks to inform and prescribe solutions and formulae to decision-makers regarding the direction and content of public policies (Weimer and Vining 1999). The purpose of policy analysis is to 'deepen, broaden and extend the policy-makers' capacity for judgement—not to provide him with answers' (Lerner 1959: 167). Political judgement can be conceptualized as using knowledge within a rationalistic model or one of a more pluralistic nature (Steinberger 1993), although with different emphases, IA (including HIA) has a place, conceptually and ontologically, within the policy analytical paradigm. Stone (2002) has produced a body of work that examines the processes of policy-making and the underlying values and politics which have an impact on the boundary and scope of policy analysis. This work examines the extent to which policy analysis can inform, objectively or subjectively (depending on which body or individual is providing the information), the public policy pathways.

Policy analysis, for the most part, refers to the analysis of policy options and alternatives. By this understanding, the type of knowledge that is fed into the policy process, and the epistemological underpinning of it (Guba and Lincoln 1989; Rossi et al. 2004), must be taken into consideration (Weiss 1977; Stone 2002). Douglas and Wildavsky (1982) conceptualize that knowledge and policy are two distinct spheres, and the two are linked by a bridge of 'information flow' which may or may not 'fit' suitably to all policy processes. It is the suitability of HIA to bridge knowledge and policy that is necessary and can result in integration. Usually, information does not find its way into policy. Weiss (1977) questioned the rationality of the linkage attributed to this information stream between policy and knowledge, stating that the values of the policy actors and researchers, and the reality of 'compromise-making' in policy processes, need to be acknowledged. Values throughout the policy process are an important consideration, whether implicit or explicit. Weiss' (1980) hypothesis is more positioned on the side of incrementalism; that policy develops as a result of 'knowledge creep' and is formulated through a process of incremental decision-making and gradual policy evolution (Bekker 2007). Indeed the rationalistic approach defies and denies the political dimension of knowledge utilization for policy. Knowledge is not often used in a non-partisan, apolitical, and technocratic manner. Oftentimes, there exists a politics of use and non-use of knowledge within the policy process; the evidence of certain knowledge put forth may be factually correct but politically inexpedient (Patton 1997). This must be taken into account in order to form an accurate picture of knowledge utilization within the public policy-making process (Chelimsky 1995).

Weiss (1991) conceptualizes this new-found land of knowledge utilization for policy as adopting a more incrementalist stance towards the domain; a long-term utilization of knowledge is incorporated into her subsequent hypothesis.

Weiss (1991) categorizes models for knowledge utilization into three groups, as cited in the work of Bekker (2007: 54/55) regarding the investigation of HIA as a tool for HPP:

1. Knowledge as a provider of facts to fill a knowledge gap.
2. Knowledge as provider of ideas for conceptual policy development.
3. Knowledge as provider of arguments as ammunition in the policy arena.

This categorization builds on the work of Janowitz (1970), who recognized the potential for conceptual utilization of knowledge over time, labelled as 'enlightenment'. The consideration of politics underlying the use of knowledge and the evaluation of policy rejects the rationalistic approach to evaluation, and recognizes the degree of policy learning that can occur in the policy processes; direct use of knowledge is no longer the only form of utilization that is recognized given the political nature of using knowledge in policy (Patton 1997; Sanderson 2002).

Rossi et al. (2004: 411) have also moved this school of thought onwards with their conceptualization and the following categorization of utilization of knowledge in policy:

1. *Instrumental utilisation:* The documented and specific use of knowledge.
2. *Conceptual utilisation:* The use of knowledge 'to influence thinking about issues in a general way'.
3. *Persuasive utilisation:* The use of knowledge 'to either support or refute political positions—in other words, to defend or attack the status quo'.

This categorization was used to establish utilization of knowledge in local policy from four completed HIAs in Northern Ireland and the Republic of Ireland. All demonstrated conceptual (indirect) utilization, whilst instrumental (direct) and persuasive (indirect) utilization were varying (O'Mullane 2009).

Such a typology was also used in the European-wide evaluation of HIA effectiveness in policy-making (Wismar et al. 2007: 19/20). Degrees of effectiveness (of use in policy) varied across the cases:

1. *Direct effectiveness:* The HIA has contributed to and modified the policy decision.
2. *General effectiveness:* The HIA was taken into consideration but the results did not modify the decision or policy.
3. *Opportunistic effectiveness:* Appears to have an effect, but in fact the HIA was only commenced because it was expected to endorse a particular policy stance.
4. *No effectiveness:* The HIA had no impact on the policy process whatsoever. No cases were categorized in this grouping.

The epistemological and ontological viewpoint of the concept 'knowledge' is a contentious point underlying the policy research of knowledge utilization: what is meant by knowledge? (Weiss 1980; Guba and Lincoln 1989; Rossi et al. 2004; Nutley et al. 2007). The meaning of knowledge is a socially constructed concept and term. The latent, and not so latent, meanings and interpretations underlying the 'knowledge' concept must be clarified at the beginning of policy processes. This point has been highlighted in the work of Bekker (2007), who investigated the policy processes and the manner in which HIAs can be redesigned to inform policy and aid decisions in the maximum way possible.

The paradigm of policy analysis, as one approach to policy study, is indeed an art and a craft, and demands the intuitive creativity and insightful foresight of practitioners, policy-makers, and researchers to 'make best use' of available knowledge for pending decisions.

Policy actors and acceptance of HIA

It is important for those involved in HIAs who occupy a position outside of the government and parliamentary circles to be mindful of the various actors within the policy space. Many policy actors have been identified in various policy studies over the past 60 years (Howlett et al. 2009). Different types of policy actors have different degrees of influence on the policy process and on policy outcomes across countries, continents, and cultures. Public policy consists of the end result of the inter-relations between the various policy actors (Howlett et al. 2009). Policy actors are not always able to act autonomously as they are often subject to the political and administrative norms and constraints within the institutions, organizations, and broader cultural frameworks within which they operate.

The range of policy actors is broad. There are many international actors such as the WHO and multilateral lending organizations such as the World Bank, the Asian Development Bank, and the African Development Bank. Domestic actors are broadly grouped into state actors (elected officials (politicians), appointed states officials), and social and political structures and actors (business actors, the labour movement, the public, research organizations, political parties, mass media, and interest or pressure groups) (Howlett et al. 2009). These groups and their influence differ across cultures, societies, institutions, countries, and continents. With regard to HIA, many originate within the public sector and public realm, and due accordance needs to be made for this with regard to public policy-making and HIA (Chilaka 2010).

The way forward for integrating HIA with the policy process

This chapter and Chapter 2 create the necessary conceptual foundation for the chapters that follow, which demonstrate the extent of an integration of HIA with the policy process, to varying degrees, using different approaches and methods. Public policy, which HIA seeks to inform with its evidence and process, in turn influences the development of HIA. IAs (including HIA) have been called policy integration tools, which are dependent on the actors and political system in which they are operating. This chapter has looked at the location of HIA within the HPP and HiAP agendas, examining instances when HIA may not the best option to take and the challenges associated with HIA and society. Policy approaches, including definitions of key terms, an overview of selected HIA policy-oriented research, and the role of a holistic approach to decision-making incorporating rationalistic and incremental leanings and a subsystems approach have been outlined. The policy cycle and its relationship with HIA have been described and the role of values in HIAs and in the policy process discussed. Policy analysis has been described, incorporating examples of HIA policy-oriented research.

The chapters that follow illustrate the resourceful and original ways in which practitioners seek to integrate HIA with the policy process. HIA has the potential to integrate as a process with the public policy processes by, for example, providing empirical data on the context of the HIA issue and generic learning points for future directions (Chapter 15), illustrating how HIA can inform national level IA processes (Chapter 7), and describing how it can integrate with other IA frameworks (Chapters 13 and 16). Although the chapters are individually focused on one country or jurisdiction at a time (apart from Chapters 4 and 5), the generic learning points at the end of each chapter exemplify the learning that can be generalized and applied across varying contexts, countries, and cultures. It is the *principle* of the learning that is important, not necessarily the geographic location. Of course, only a portion of the global activity of integrating HIA is represented here. What is presented and shared in this book is a variety of ways to integrate HIA with the policy process, in order to inspire and urge us onwards to embrace and develop HIA as an instrument and approach that *can* better inform the policy processes of health impacts.

Acknowledgements

The author would like to acknowledge the invaluable input of Patrick Harris to this chapter.

Bibliography

Abdel-Aziz, M.I., Radford, J., and McCabe, J. (2004) The Finningley Airport Health Impact Assessment: A Case Study, in Kemm, J., Parry, J., and Palmer, S. (eds), *Health Impact Assessment: Concepts, Theories, Techniques and Applications*. Oxford: Oxford University Press.

Ahmad, B., Chappel, D., Pless-Mulloli, T., White, M. (2008) Enabling factors and barriers for the use of health impact assessment in decision-making processes. *Public Health* 122: 452–457.

Atkinson, P. and Cooke, A. (2005) Developing a Framework to Assess the Costs and Benefits of Health Impact Assessment. *Environmental Impact Assessment Review* 25: 791–798.

Banken, R. (2001) *Strategies for Institutionalising HIA*. Brussels: European Centre for Health Policy.

Bekker, M. (2007) *The Politics of Healthy Policies: Redesigning HIA to Integrate Health in Public Policy, Postbus*. The Netherlands: Eburon Delft.

Bekker, M.P.M., Putters, K., and Van der Grinten, T.E.D. (2004) Exploring the relations between evidence and decision-making: A political-administrative approach to health impact assessment. *Environmental Impact Assessment Review* 24: 139–149.

Bhatia, R. and Corburn, J. (2011) Lessons from San Francisco: Health Impact Assessments Have Advanced Political Conditions for Improving Population Health. *Health Affairs* 30 (12): 2410–2418.

Birley, M.H. (2011) *Health Impact Assessment: Principles and Practice*. London: Earthscan.

Birley, M.H. and Peralta, G.L. (1992) *Guidelines for the health impact assessment of development projects*. Asian Development Bank Environmental Paper no 11. Manila: Asian Development Bank.

Cashmore, M., Richardson, T., Hilding-Ryedvik, T., and Emmelin, L. (2010) Evaluating the effectiveness of impact assessment instruments: theorising the nature and implications of their political constitution. *Environmental Impact Assessment Review* 30: 371–379.

Chelimsky, E. (1995) Where we stand today in the practice of evaluation: Some reflections. *Knowledge and Policy* 8 (3): 8–20.

Chilaka, M.A. (2010) Vital statistics relating to the practice of health impact assessment (HIA) in the United Kingdom. *Environmental Impact Assessment Review* 30: 116–119.

Close, N. (2001) *Alconbury Airfield Development Health Impact Assessment Evaluation Report*. Cambridge: Cambridgeshire Health Authority.

Collins, J. and Koplan, J.P. (2009) Health impact assessment: a step toward health in all policies. *Journal of the American Medical Association* 302: 315–317.

Dannenberg, A.L., Bhatia, R., Cole, B.L., Heaton, S.K., Feldman, J.D., and Rutt, C.D. (2008) Use of health impact assessment in the US: 27 case studies, 1999–2007. *American Journal of Preventive Medicine* 34 (3): 241–256.

Dannenberg, A.L., Frumkin, H., and Jackson, R.J. (2011) *Making healthy places: designing and building for health, well-being and sustainability*. Washington: Island Press.

Davenport, C., Mathers, J., and Parry, J. (2006) Use of health impact assessment in incorporating health considerations in decision making. *Journal of Epidemiology and Community Health* 60: 196–201.

Douglas, M. and Wildavsky, A. (1982) *Risk and Culture*. Berkley: University of California Press.

Dye, T.R. (1976) *What Governments Do, Why They Do It, What Difference It Makes*. Alabama: Alabama University Press.

Easton, D. (1953) *The Political System*. New York: Knopf.

Elliott, E. and Francis, S. (2005) Making effective links to decision-making: key challenges for health impact assessment. *Environmental Impact Assessment Review* 25 (7–8): 747–757.

Elliott, E. and Williams, G. (2008) Developing public sociology through health impact assessment. *Sociology of Health and Illness* 30 (7): 1–16.

Etzioni, A. (1967) Mixed-scanning: a 'third' approach to decision-making. *Public Administration Review*, 27: 385–392

Fox, D. (2012) *Towards a framework for evaluating the role of impact assessment in promoting social and environmental justice: a pilot study of health impact assessment*. PhD thesis. Liverpool: University of Liverpool.

Gagnon, F., Turgeon, J., and Dallaire, C. (2007) Healthy public policy: a conceptual cognitive framework. *Health Policy* 81 (1): 42–55.

Guba, E.G. and Lincoln, Y.S. (1989) *Fourth Generation Evaluation*. Newbury Park, CA: Sage Publications.

Ham, C. and Hill, M. (1993) *The Policy Process in the Modern Capitalist State*, 2nd edn. London: Harvester Wheatsheaf.

Haigh, F., Harris, P., and Haigh, N. (2012) Health impact assessment research and practice: a place for paradigm positioning? *Environment Impact Assessment Review* 33 (1): 66–72.

Harris-Roxas, B. and Harris, E. (in press) The impact and effectiveness of health impact assessment: a conceptual framework. *Environmental Impact Assessment Review*.

Harris, P., Sainsbury, P., and Kemp, L. (2012) *HIA and Public Policy Internationally: Essential Elements for Sustaining HIA, Plenary Session 'How to make HIA stick'*. Inaugural National Health Impact Assessment Meeting, 3–4 April, Washington DC.

Harris, P. (forthcoming thesis) The relationship between HIA and HPP Sydney: Centre for Health Equity Training Research and Evaluation, University of New South Wales.

Harris, P. (2012) Personal correspondence, 8th July 2012.

Harris-Roxas, B., Viliani, F., Harris, P., Bond, A., Cave, B., Divall, M., Furu, P., Soeberg, M., Wernham, A., and Winkler, M. (2012) Health impact assessment: the state of the art. *Impact Assessment and Project Appraisal* 1: 1–11.

Heclo, H. (1972) Review Article: Policy analysis. *British Journal of Political Science* 2: 83–108.

Hogwood, B.W. and Gunn, L.A. (1984) *Policy Analysis for the Real World*. Oxford: Oxford University Press.

Howlett, M., Ramesh, M., and Perl, A. (2009) *Studying Public Policy: Policy Cycles and Policy Subsystems*. Oxford: Oxford University Press.

International Finance Corporation (2009) *Introduction to Health Impact Assessment*. Washington, DC: International Finance Corporation.

Jackson, R., Bear, D., Bhatia, R., Cantor, S.B., Cave, B., Diez Roux, A.V., Dora, C., Fielding, J.E., Zivin, J.S.G., Levy, J.I., Quint, J.I., Raja, S., Schulz, A.J., and Wernham, A.A. (2011) *Improving Health in the United States: the Role of Health Impact Assessment*.

Washington DC: Committee on Health Impact Assessment, National Research Council of the National Academies. Available at <http://www.nap.edu/catalog.php?record_id=13229>. Accessed 5 July 2012.

Janowitz, M. (1970) *Political Conflict: Essays in Political Sociology*. Chicago: Quadrangle Books.

Jasonoff, S. (2004) *Design on Nature: Science and Democracy in Europe and the United States*. Princeton: Princeton University Press.

John, P. (1998) *Analysing Public Policy*. London and New York: Continuum.

Jordan, A. and O' Riordan, T. (2001) Environmental politics and policy processes, in O'Riordan, T. (ed.), *Environmental Science for Environmental Management*. Harlow: Prentice-Hall.

Kearns, N. and Pursell, L. (2007) *Evaluation of the HIA of Traffic and Transport in Ballyfermot*. Galway: Department of Health Promotion, Galway: National University of Ireland.

Kearns, N. and Pursell, L. (2011) Time for a paradigm change? Tracing the institutionalisation of health impact assessment in the Republic of Ireland across health and environmental sectors. *Health Policy* 99 (2): 91–96.

Kemm, J. (2001) Health impact assessment: a tool for healthy public policy. *Health Promotion International* 16 (1): 79–85.

Kemm, J. (2005) The future challenges for HIA. *Environmental Impact Assessment Review* 25: 799–807.

Kemm, J. (2006) Past and Future of Health Impact Assessment. Comprehensive Health Impact Assessment Training Course, 25–27 September. Dublin: Institute of Public Health.

Kemm, J. (2011) HIA-advocacy or impartiality. 11th HIA International Conference, Granada, 14–15 April.

Kemm, J. and Parry, J. (2004) What is health impact assessment? Introduction and overview, in Kemm, J., Parry, J., and Palmer, S. (eds), *Health Impact Assessment: Concepts, Theories, Techniques and Applications,* pp. 1–14. Oxford: Oxford University Press.

Kemm, J., den Broeder, L., Wismar, M., Fehr, R., Douglas, M., and Guliš, G. (2011) *How can HIA support Health in All Policies*? Draft document presented at the Poznan Meeting of Polish EU Presidency, 8 November 2011.

Knoepfel, P., Larrue, C., Varone, F., and Hill, M. (2007) *Public Policy Analysis*. Bristol: Policy Press.

Knol, A.B., Briggs, D.J., and Lebret, E. (2010) Assessment of complex environmental health problems: framing the structures and structuring the frameworks. *Science of the Total Environment* 408: 2785–2794.

Krieger, N., Northridge, M., Gruskin, S., Quinn, M., Kriebel, D., Davey-Smith, G., Bassett, M., Rehkopf, D.H., and Millar, C. (2003) Assessing health impact assessment: multidisciplinary and international perspectives. *Journal of Epidemiology and Community Health* 57: 659–662.

Lasswell, H. (1935) *Politics: Who gets what, when, how*. London: McGraw-Hill.

Lasswell, H.D. (1956) The Political Science of Science: An Inquiry into the Possible Reconciliation of Mastery and Freedom. *American Political Review* 50 (4): 961–979.

Lasswell, H.D. (1959) Strategies of Enquiry: The Rational Use of Observation, in Lerner, D. (ed.), *The Human Meaning of the Social Sciences*. New York: Meridian Books.

Lindblom, C.E. and Woodhouse, E.J. (1993) *The Policy-Making Process*, 3rd edition. New Jersey: Prentice-Hall.

Mahoney, M. (2009) Imperatives for Policy Health Impact Assessment: perspectives, positions, power relations. Unpublished PhD thesis, Deakin University.

Mathias, K. and Harris-Roxas, B. (2009) Process and impact evaluation of the Greater Christchurch Urban Development Strategy Health Impact Assessment. *BioMed Central Public Health* 9: 97.

Metcalfe, O. and Higgins, C. (2009) Healthy public policy—is health impact assessment the cornerstone? *Public Health* 123: 296–301.

Milio, N. (1981) *Promoting Health through Public Policy*. Philadelphia: FA Davis.

Lerner, D (1959) *The Human Meaning of the Social Sciences*. New York: Meridian Books.

Milner, S.J., Bailey, C., and Deans, J. (2003) Fit for purpose health impact assessment: a realistic way forward. *Public Health* 117 (5): 295–300.

Mindell, J., Hansell, A., Morrison, D., Douglas, M., and Joffe, M. (2001) What do we need for robust, quantitative health impact assessment? *Journal of Public Health Medicine* 23(3): 173–178.

Morgan, G. (2009) On the limitations of health impact assessment. *Public Health* 123 (12): 820.

Nutley, S.M., Walter, I., and Davies, H.T.O. (2007) *Using Evidence: How Research can Inform Public Services*. Bristol: The Policy Press.

O'Faircheallaigh, C. (2009) Public policy processes and sustainability in the minerals and energy industries, in Richards, J. (ed.), *Mining, Society, and a Sustainable World*, pp. 437–467. Berlin, Heidelberg: Springer.

O'Mullane, M. (2009) *An investigation of the utilisation of health impact assessments (HIAs) in Irish public policy making*. PhD thesis. Cork: University College Cork.

O'Mullane, M. and Quinlivan, A. (2012) Health impact assessment (HIA) in Ireland and the role of local government. *Environmental Impact Assessment Review* 32: 181–186.

Organization for African Unity (1997) Harare declaration on malaria prevention and control in the context of African economic recovery and development. Organization of African Unity Assembly of Heads of State and Government, 33rd Ordinary Session, AHG/Decl 1 XXXIII, 2–4 June. Available at <http://www.iss.co.za/AF/RegOrg/unity_to_union/pdfs/oau/hog/7HoG ssembly1997>.pdf. Accessed 6 June 2012.

Parry, J.M. and Stevens, A.J. (2001) Prospective health impact assessment: problems, pitfalls and possible ways forward. *British Medical Journal* 323: 1177–1182.

Parry, J. and Wright, J. (2003) Community participation in health impact assessments: intuitively appealing but practically difficult. *Bulletin of the World Health Organization* 55: 219–220.

Patton, M.Q. (1997) *Utilisation-Focused Evaluation, Thousand Oaks*, 3rd edition. California: Sage Publications.

Petticrew, M., Whitehead, M., Macintyre, S.J., Graham, H., and Egan, M. (2004) Evidence for public health policy on inequalities 1: the reality according to policy-makers, *Journal of Epidemiology and Community Health* 58: 811–816.

Putters, K. (2005) Health impact assessment, the next step: defining models and roles. *Environmental Impact Assessment Review* 25: 693–701.

Quigley, R.J. and Taylor, L.C. (2003) evaluation as a key part of health impact assessment: the English experience. *Bulletin of the World Health Organization* 81 (3): 415–419.

Quigley, R. J. and Taylor, L.C. (2004) Evaluating health impact assessment. *Public Health* 118: 544–552.

Rossi, P.H., Lipsey, M.W., and Freeman, H.E. (2004) *Evaluation: A Systematic Approach*, 7th edition. Thousand Oaks, CA: Sage Publications.

Sabatier, P.A. (1999) *Theories of the Policy Process*. Boulder, CO: Westview Press.

Sanderson, I. (2002) Evaluation, policy learning and evidence-based policy-making. *Public Administration* 80 (1): 1–22.

Scott-Samuel, A. (2006) *Forum Chair: Healthy Public Policy*. 7th International Health Impact Assessment Conference, Cardiff, 5–6 April.

Steinberger, P.J. (1993) *The Concept of Political Judgement*. Chicago and London: University of Chicago Press.

Stone, D. (2002) *Policy Paradox: The Art of Political Decision Making*. New York: W.W. Norton.

St-Pierre, L. (2007), 'HIA and the Practices of Public Health Actors in Support of Healthy Public Policies,' 8th International HIA Conference, *Healthy Public Policies- Is HIA the Cornerstone*? Dublin Castle, Ireland, 16th–17th October.

Taylor, L. and Blair-Stevens, C. (2002) *Introducing Health Impact Assessment: Informing the Decision-Making Process*. London: Health Development Agency.

Walt, G. (1994) *Health Policy: An Introduction to Process and Power*. London: Zed Books.

Weimer, D.L. and Vining, A.R. (1999) *Policy Analysis: Concepts and Practice*, 3rd edn. New Jersey: Prentice Hall.

Weiss, C.H. (1977) *Using Social Research in Public Policy-Making*. Policy Studies Organisation Series. Toronto: Lexington Books.

Weiss, C.H. (1980) Knowledge creep and decision accretion. *Knowledge: Creation, Diffusion, Utilisation* 1(3): 381–404.

Weiss, C.H. (1991) Policy research: data, ideas or arguments? in Wagner, P., Weiss, C.H., Wittrock, B., and Wollman, H. (eds), *Social Sciences and Modern States: National Experiences and Theoretical Crossroads*. Cambridge: Cambridge University Press.

Wendel, A., Dannenberg, A., and Frumkin, H. (2008) Designing and building healthy places for children. *International Journal for Environment and Health* 2 (3/4): 338–355.

WHO (1999) *Health Impact Assessment: Main Concepts and Suggested Approach*. Gothenburg Consensus Paper. Brussels: WHO.

WHO (1986) *Ottawa Charter for Health Promotion*. Geneva: WHO.

WHO (2012) *The role of HIA in decision making*. Geneva: WHO. Available at <http://www.who.int/hia/policy/decision/en/index.html>. Accessed 6 July 2012.

Wildavsky, A.B. (1979) *Speaking Truth to Power: The Art and Craft of Policy Analysis*. Boston: Little Brown.

Wismar, M., Blau, J., Ernst, K., and Figueras, J. (2007) Implementing and institutional-izing health impact assessment in Europe, in Wismar, M., Blau, J., Ernst, K., and Figueras, J. (eds), *The Effectiveness of Health Impact Assessment: Scope and Limitations of Supporting Decision-making in Europe*, pp. 57–78. Copenhagen: European Observatory on Health Systems and Policies, WHO.

Chapter 4

The impact of health impact assessment on the policy-making process in Ireland: Northern Ireland and the Republic of Ireland

Claire Higgins, Owen Metcalfe,
and Noëlle Cotter

Introduction

Public health challenges facing the island of Ireland include an ageing population, a predicted rise in chronic conditions, an obesity epidemic, and specific public health concerns such as suicide and alcohol-related deaths. Since 1998, the Institute of Public Health in Ireland (IPH) has been working to improve cooperation for public health on the island of Ireland and tackle these issues.

Better decision-making for better health occurs when there is greater awareness of the factors that influence health together with the capacity and willingness to influence decisions in favour of health. IPH supports better decision-making for better health by improving the quality of, and access to, health intelligence, and providing policy advice and building capacity in agencies, organizations, and government departments at all levels.

From a policy perspective IPH derives support for health impact assessment (HIA) in Northern Ireland (NI) through the *Investing for Health* strategy, which refers to HIA as a key tool to facilitate cross-sectoral action and a means to promote health and reduce inequalities (Department of Health, Social Services and Public Safety 2002). In the Republic of Ireland (RoI), policy commitments and objectives for HIA are included in a number of documents, including the health strategy *Quality and Fairness: A health system for you*, which states that HIA is expected to play an important role in promoting a joint approach as it is a means for all sectors to determine effects and actions on health (Department of Health and Children 2001).

Both NI and RoI have experienced major changes to health system administration over the last decade. The establishment of the Public Health Agency (PHA) in NI and the Health Service Executive (HSE) in the RoI represent opportunities to progress HIA and identify it as an important way to contribute to collaborative working for improved health.

IPH believes a health in all policies (HiAP) approach must be adopted and to facilitate this has given priority to developing capacity to undertake and engage in HIA in line with international practice (Quigley 2010). A focus of all IPH work is tackling health inequalities and HIA has proven valuable in this context as it allows for a systematic assessment of the distributive effects of the policy, programme, or project on subgroups of the population. IPH work in HIA has concentrated on:

◆ capacity building, which includes awareness raising, training, and networking

◆ undertaking and contributing to HIAs

◆ contributing to the evidence base with literature reviews to support more informed decision-making.

(Metcalfe and Higgins 2009)

Embedding at strategic policy and structural levels demonstrates an increasing recognition of HIA potential. However, a considerable time lag exists in implementing HIA across health and environment policy areas, both of which have been given clear strategic remits for HIA at the macro-level, particularly in the RoI (Kearns and Pursell 2011).

The island of Ireland remains at an early stage of HIA implementation and it is clear that policies, systems, and structures exist to facilitate HIA. A core challenge that remains is the translation of policy intentions into practice. A major paradigm change is required in order to facilitate systematic commitment to HIA within a relevant organizational structure at both meso and micro levels. The importance of institutional culture and political will are key factors in the implementation process (Kearns and Pursell 2011).

The case studies that follow are illustrative of HIAs undertaken in NI and the RoI, demonstrating contributions to tackling inequalities and a move to more effective decision-making processes to improve health.

Case study: Northern Ireland

Health impact assessment of the Service Framework for Cardiovascular Health and Wellbeing

Background

The concept of service frameworks was introduced by the Chief Medical Officer in 2007 to improve health and social care outcomes, reduce inequities in health and wellbeing, and enhance service access and delivery in NI. Service frameworks set out standards and performance measures for health and social care service providers in relation to prevention, diagnosis, treatment, rehabilitation, and palliative care in individuals and communities, making clear statements about what types and levels of service should be available to service users and aiming for integration of services along care pathways.

Cardiovascular disease (CVD) includes heart disease, stroke, and other circulation problems, and is impacted by conditions such as obesity, diabetes, and blood lipid disorders. CVD remains the main cause of death and disability in NI and despite improvements over many years is still a major contributor to health inequalities (Department of Health, Social Services and Public Safety 2009).

The 'substantial excess burden of morbidity and mortality due to cardiovascular disease in disadvantaged groups raises major challenges' (Capewell and Graham 2010: 1). In NI, men living in the least deprived areas live on average 8 years longer than men in the most deprived areas and for women this gap is 5 years.

It is a common misconception that health policies do not require HIA because of their nature of improving health. In this circumstance HIA was undertaken to strengthen the implementation of the Service Framework for Cardiovascular Health and Wellbeing (CVSFW) in relation to tackling health inequalities and inequities, and to demonstrate how HIA can provide a useful process to support commissioning for equitable health and social care services.

The PHA is leading the implementation of the CVSFW and in accordance with its corporate aim to reduce health inequalities, identified HIA as a way to test the potential impact of CVSFW standard implementation on health inequalities and inequities. Outputs from the HIA would inform and contribute to the annual health and social care (HSC) business plan and mid-term review of the CVSFW scheduled for 2012. This approach is in line with recommended good practice from the National Institute for Health and Clinical Excellence (NICE), who advocate HIA for the assessment of policies on cardiovascular disease and the potential impact on health inequalities (NICE 2010). Learning from the HIA could be applied to other service frameworks to ensure unintended effects, especially on health inequalities and inequities, would be minimized or avoided in other policy areas.

Using HIA to support policy implementation

To assess the health impacts of CVSFW standard implementation, information was collected in four ways. The wider policy context was interpreted whilst the community profile presented a picture of cardiovascular health and its determinants in NI. A literature review considered published evidence on effective interventions to improve cardiovascular health and wellbeing. A desktop appraisal tool, developed by an external expert HIA advisor, was used to guide consultation with and engagement of people in community and statutory sectors in a series of workshops (Figure 4.1).

Potential impacts on health inequalities and health inequities:
• Are there any pre-existing health inequalities associated with this standard?
• Are there any inequities in health associated with this standard?
Potential barriers to realising the standard's intended impacts on health
• Are there any barriers to the implementation of the standard as a whole?
• Are there any barriers to the implementation of one or more of the actions contained within the standard?
Potential impacts on health services
• Will the implementation of the standard affect demand for the services described in the standard?
• Will the implementation of the standard affect need for health and social care services in future?
• How will the implementation of the standard affect staff responsible for delivering the services described in the standard?
Potential impacts of the implementation of the standard on health and wellbeing
Potential impacts of the implementation of the standard on health inequalities and inequities
Potential impacts of the implementation of the standard on the determinants of health
How can we enhance any positive effects of the standard and its implementation, including ways to reduce health inequalities and/or health inequities?
How can we minimise or avoid any unintended negative effects of the standard and its implementation, including those that could exacerbate health inequalities and/or health inequities?

Fig. 4.1 Desktop appraisal tool. Developed by Erica Ison, specialist practitioner in HIA, affiliated to the Public Health Resource Unit Oxford. Reproduced with permission of the developer.

Analysis of the desktop appraisal findings provided understanding as to how each of the 45 CVSFW standards were likely to impact on health inequalities and inequities if implemented. Suggestions were sought on how to improve health outcomes through CVSFW standard implementation, and identify and avoid unintended adverse effects on health equality and equity of service provision. Barriers to the implementation of each standard and ways to overcome them were also identified. These related to the capacity of systems, organizations, and staff to facilitate and support change.

Numerous suggestions were generated that required prioritization along a set of agreed criteria. These included:

◆ the number of people affected
◆ the expected impact on health inequalities and inequities
◆ evidence of effectiveness
◆ timescale

A weighted health action plan containing suggestions for each of the CVSFW standards was developed.

A formal evaluation has not been undertaken yet, but the impact of the HIA and its contribution to health and social care delivery is evident.

The impact on policy-making

This work emphasizes the importance of considering impacts of health policy design and implementation on health inequalities and inequities. It has increased awareness of HIA as a policy assessment tool and equipped many staff in HSC organizations with skills to undertake HIA. This process has provided deeper understanding of what HSC services can and need to do to reduce health inequalities and enabled people to use their knowledge and expertise to contribute to discussions on how to improve service delivery (PHA 2011). The HIA determined that the CVSFW will make a positive contribution towards improving health equity.

All of this is taking place in a period of severe financial constraints and difficult decisions are being made in relation to funding HSC services. This case study shows how HIA can provide a framework for determining how services might impact on health inequalities and inequities beyond the assumption that HSC policies and service development are good for health.

Beyond these considerations of socio-economic sustainability for HSC services, the HIA highlighted the importance of being able to collect, analyse, and interpret HSC usage and outcome data in ways that allow disaggregation of information by socio-economic markers of relevant populations. Policy decisions are required to move away from global activity measures and target setting for HSC services towards more sophisticated and meaningful ways of assessing the performance and outcomes of HSC service provision for distinct population groups.

This case study demonstrates the relevance of and need to conduct HIA on health service policies and presents a mechanism to influence and direct the commissioning of services and implementation of the CVSFW. It provides an example of how HSC considered the potential impacts of its work and demonstrates how the delivery of policy can impact on health inequalities and inequities. The HIA of the CVSFW has also demonstrated that, unintentionally, HSC policies can have adverse impacts on health equity and provides a methodology to identify and mitigate these to reduce health inequalities. It has also raised awareness of health inequalities and inequities across a wide range of people from different sectors.

Much of the success of this work can be attributed to applying a rigorous approach to collecting information for the HIA. The thorough appraisal design allowed interpretation of consultation outputs and other information sources to provide insights into and evidence for a focus on HSC service development that strengthens the effort to reduce health inequalities.

Case study: Republic of Ireland

Limerick regeneration health impact assessment

Background

Limerick city is one of the RoI's larger urban centres. It has attracted undesirable media attention over the last decade due to significant criminality and antisocial behaviour, in particular centred on the Moyross housing estate to the north of the city. Criminal activity and serious social problems became synonymous with the area, and the tipping point was reached in September 2006 when two children were seriously injured when the car they were in was petrol-bombed. The national outcry resulting from this incident led the government to undertake an investigation of the issues prevailing in this area and make recommendations directly to the Cabinet Committee on Social Inclusion. From the outset, therefore, the problems associated with this area were embedded in a discourse of social exclusion rather than focused on associated outcomes such as criminality alone. The report to the Cabinet had three strands:

◆ dealing with criminality—seen as fundamental to creating the conditions for other interventions to be successful and for restoring the confidence of local communities
◆ economic and infrastructural regeneration—to create employment, unlock value, improve access, and achieve a better commercial and housing mix
◆ develop coordinated responses to social and educational problems to break the cycle of disadvantage.

The Fitzgerald Report (2007) to the Cabinet Committee in terms of methodology particularly embraced the need to engage with the community for a 'bottom-up' approach. In addition, it recognized the need for interagency working and communication as essential to an effective process. From the outset there were parallels with HIA paradigms: understanding the determinants and causality of social outcomes, the influence of sectors on each other's agendas, and the importance of community engagement and empowerment.

A key element of the Report's recommendations was to create two special-purpose agencies for the south and north of Limerick city. The Limerick Regeneration Agencies' objective is to improve the quality of life for residents within key Limerick city locations through the creation and implementation of a programme that will incorporate quality-designed modern homes, improved community facilities, and integrated services.

Using HIA to support policy implementation

The HSE local health promotion team was the driver behind the Regeneration Agencies undertaking three HIAs on the following elements of the regeneration process:

◆ physical regeneration
◆ early school leaving, absenteeism, and truancy
◆ integrated youth space(s)

These three were chosen as the physical regeneration proposals were swiftly progressing, while the topic of young people consistently arose during consultation and therefore dealing with young people's issues was appropriate to address multiple agendas.

Physical regeneration

The HIA physical regeneration recommendations are included in the Implementation Plan, demonstrating the gravitas afforded for the HIA process and the alignment of the HIA outcomes with thinking already undertaken by project overseers. The Physical Regeneration Plan, in terms of housing, centres on the idea of providing mixed tenure to include housing under the Affordable Homes Scheme (see <http://www.housing.ie> for more information on this scheme). However, given the collapse of the property market that has occurred in the RoI since 2008, this scheme is now largely redundant and indeed attracting private households for purchase of new units may also prove difficult. The commercial aspect of the physical regeneration is reliant on public–private partnerships. These are unlikely to proceed in the current climate in spite of suggested tax incentives, which may no longer be viable. The HIA was used constructively to influence the physical redesign elements and demonstrates the openness of the Regeneration Plan to take on board recommendations for improved health.

Early school leaving, absenteeism, and truancy

This HIA identified the general needs in the area with particular emphasis on early years interventions, retention into post-primary education, and adult education and training. However, the focus was particularly on changing national level policies and this could be seen as beyond the remit of the regeneration process. Many of the more specific recommendations are addressed in the subsequent *Limerick Regeneration Programme 2009–2018* (the masterplan; Limerick Regeneration Agencies 2008) with regard to providing educational opportunities in the area. However, the emphasis on increasing graduate numbers and training opportunities, and the economic rationale for this is repeated throughout. In August 2010 there were 60,000 unemployed graduates in the RoI (Duncan 2010) and improved educational opportunities may not have immediate tangible beneficial outcomes for people in the locality.

Integrated youth space

The integrated youth space implemented all the HIA recommendations that were highly specific and practical. This could be attributed to the fact that an integrated youth space is a smaller self-contained project within the regeneration process and in addition the presence of youth workers at a grassroots level ensured this project was prioritized. The aforementioned HIAs were less specific in their recommendations, which paralleled the embryonic stage in the process that the regeneration was at; the intent was to carry the HIA process through the development of the regeneration project. This process may have benefited from HIA as an integrated, targeted, and ongoing element to the project with an ability to critique specific proposals as they arose, while also addressing the new economic realities and changing circumstances.

The impact on policy-making in relation to local regeneration

This case study shows that overall the HIA processes appear to have made positive contributions to the development of the regeneration plans, and the principles underscoring HIA similarly underpinned the thinking behind the Fitzgerald Report and masterplan. However, Limerick Regeneration faces an uphill struggle given the current economic climate and austere policy context. Indicative of the struggle facing Limerick, a report by Fahey et al. (2011) concluded that the significant financial investment during the boom era appeared to make little impact on the area. What we must now hope is that the HIA process, with its emphasis on community development approaches coupled with the considerable community solidarity that exists, will support and progress these projects, albeit in a different manner to that envisaged when significant financial investment was available.

Generic learning points

These two HIA case studies present different approaches to HIA. In them the health sector was the driving force for championing the health agenda in two very different scenarios.

REFERENCES | 53

For public health practitioners and policy-makers

- From a practitioners perspective it is evident IPH played a role in developing capacity for HIA across the island of Ireland. Champions in HIA referred to in this chapter attended HIA training hosted by IPH, who were central to supporting both case studies.

- Central to influencing policies is coordinated institutional action. These case studies demonstrate the importance of identifying and working with stakeholders from all sectors for improved health outcomes, which was particularly evident in the approach to the HIA in Limerick.

- Providing training for HIA is not sufficient on its own but putting theory into practice requires support, direction, and guidance alongside a suite of tools and sufficient resources to secure implementation. IPH has developed a package of support mechanisms but greater championing for HIA in sectors outside health is still required in the policy-making process to truly deliver on an HiAP agenda.

For educators and researchers

- It is clear that HIA is a tool to support placing an emphasis on health inequalities and inequities in healthcare planning and delivery. It provides a structured framework for taking action. HIA has shown how a health agenda aligns with a drive to regenerate a disadvantaged area to improve living conditions and health outcomes.

- Timing is crucial to the HIA being able to influence the policy decision. However, external factors, as indicated in the Limerick Regeneration case study, clearly highlight the wider political, social, and economic context within which HIA operates and more importantly needs to take account of. In the CVSFW case study timing was crucial to ensure suggestions were incorporated in the business planning activities.

- The case studies demonstrate how recommendations that are more focused and specific may be integrated more readily than those seeking to address national level policy.

References

Capewell, S. and Graham, H. (2010) Will cardiovascular disease prevention widen health inequalities? PLOS Medicine 7 (8): 1–8.
Department of Health and Children (2001) *Quality and Fairness—A Health System for You*. Dublin: Department of Health and Children.
Department of Health, Social Services and Public Safety (2002) *Investing for Health*. Belfast: Department of Health, Social Services and Public Safety.

Department of Health, Social Services and Public Safety (2009) *Service Framework for Cardiovascular Health and Wellbeing.* Available at <http://www.dhsspsni.gov.uk/showconsultations?txtid=30036>. Accessed 21 July 2011.

Duncan, P. (2010) 'Graduate options: slim to none'. *The Irish Times*, 8 August. Available at <http://www.irishtimes.com/newspaper/weekend/2010/0814/1224276782623.html>. Accessed 19 August 2010.

Fahey, T., Norris, M., McCafferty, D., and Humphreys, E. (2011) *Combating Social Disadvantage in Social Housing Estates: The policy implications of a ten-year follow-up study.* Combat Poverty Agency Working Paper Series 11/02. Available at <http://www.cpa.ie/publications/workingpapers/2011–02_WP_CombatingSocialDisadvantageInSocialHousingEstates.pdf>. Accessed 19 September 2012.

Fitzgerald Report (2007) *Addressing Issues of Social Exclusion in Moyross and Other Disadvantaged Areas of Limerick City: Report to the Cabinet Committee on Social Exclusion.* Available at <http://www.limerickregeneration.ie/wp-content/uploads/2008/10/social_inclusion_limerick.pdf>. Accessed 29 August 2011.

Kearns, N. and Pursell, L. (2011) Time for a paradigm change? Tracing the institutionalisation of health impact assessment in the Republic of Ireland across health and environmental sectors. *Health Policy* 99: 91–96.

Limerick Regeneration Agencies (2008) *The Limerick Regeneration Programme 2009–2018.* Available at <http://www.limerickregeneration.ie/plans-index/>. Accessed 29 August 2011.

Metcalfe, O. and Higgins, C. (2009) Healthy public policy: is health impact assessment the cornerstone? *Public Health* 123 (4): 296–301.

NICE (2010) *Prevention of cardiovascular disease.* Available at <http://guidance.nice.org.uk/PH25>. Accessed 14 June 2011.

PHA (2011) *Putting a health inequalities focus on the northern ireland cardiovascular service framework: Technical report.* Available at <http://www.publichealth.hscni.net/publications/putting-health-inequalities-focus-northern-ireland-cardiovascular-service-framework>. Accessed 21 July 2011.

Quigley, R. (2010) Role of health impact assessment in health in all policies, in Kickbusch, I. and Buckett, K. (eds) *Implementing Health in All Policies: Adelaide 2010.* Government of South Australia. Available at <http://www.sahealth.sa.gov.au/wps/wcm/connect/0ab5f18043aee450b600feed1a914d95/implementinghiapadel-sahealth-100622.pdf?MOD=AJPERES&CACHEID=0ab5f18043aee450b600feed1a914d95>. Accessed 25 July 2011.

Chapter 5

Health impact assessment implementation and public health policy systems in Denmark and Slovakia

Gabriel Guliš and Jana Kollárová

Introduction

Denmark and Slovakia are of similar geographic size and total population (WHO HFA (Health for All) 2012), but have different historical and political development. Differences in history and politics provided a different context for the development of public health systems in the two countries. Major political, demographic, and socio-economic information as well as historical development milestones of both countries are presented in Table 5.1.

The Danish population enjoys a longer life expectancy with slightly lower differences between men and women; the percentage of elderly is higher in Denmark. Both countries are members of the European Union (EU); Denmark is considered one of the 'traditional' EU countries. Slovakia is a very young state and democracy; the country was established on 1 January 1993 and joined the EU within the group of 10 new member states in 2004. Both countries are governed by a parliamentary democracy system; in the case of Denmark, along with a constitutional monarchy system. Probably for historical reasons, the Danish system is more decentralized than the Slovak one: health issues on a national level are part of the agenda of the Danish Ministry of Health and Prevention supported by the National Board of Health, and most of the practical activities are in the regional (health care) or local (public health/health promotion) level. Slovakia has a Ministry of Health that oversees the Public Health Authority of the Slovak Republic and a network of 36 regional public health authorities in accordance with 79 districts. Both countries (Denmark in 1989 and the Slovak Republic in 1994) implemented environmental impact

Table 5.1 Basic information on Denmark and Slovakia

Indicator	Denmark	Slovak Republic	Reference
Geographic area (km²)	43,075	49,035	WHO HFA 2012
Population (2011 estimate)	5,560,628	5,435,273	WHO HFA 2012
% of population aged 65+ (2005)	15.11	11.74	WHO HFA 2012
Life expectancy at birth (males/females) in 2009	76.9/81.1	71.4/79.1	WHO HFA 2012
Infant mortality	4.43 (2005)*	5.86 (2007)**	*WHO HFA 2012 **Health Statistics 2007
Total unemployment rate (May 2011)	7.4	13.3	Eurostat 2011
Unemployment rates of the population aged 25–64 by level of education: pre-primary, primary and lower secondary education	8.6	40.8	Eurostat 2011
Unemployment rates of the population aged 25–64 by level of education: upper secondary and post-secondary non-tertiary education	6.2	12.3	Eurostat 2011
Unemployment rates of the population aged 25–64 by level of education: tertiary education	4.8	4.9	Eurostat 2011
Political system	Parliamentary democracy and constitutional monarchy	Parliamentary democracy	
Governance levels	Three (national, regional, local)	Three (national, regional, local)	
Health system	Public funding via taxation with a certain level of private system supported by private insurance, Ministry of Health and Prevention	Public funding via health insurance with a certain level of private system supported by private insurance, Ministry of Health	

(*continued*)

Table 5.1 (*Continued*)

Indicator	Denmark	Slovak Republic	Reference
Membership of European Union	1973	2004	
GDP per capita in PPS (EU-27 = 100) (2010)	124	74	WHO HFA 2012
UNDP Human development index (2007)	0.955	0.88	WHO HFA 2012
Other impact assessments	EIA, HTA, SEA	EIA, SEA, HTA beginning	

assessment (EIA) and signed the Protocol on strategic environmental assessment (SEA). In Denmark there is a relatively large network of experts and institutions for health technology assessment (HTA); in Slovakia HTA is only just beginning. The centralized (top-down) versus decentralized (bottom-up) type of governance predetermines the expected method of implementation of health impact assessment (HIA) in both countries. The public health systems, as potential leaders for HIA implementation, are described in more detail in the following section.

Public health systems of Denmark and the Slovak Republic

Table 5.2 provides basic information on these two public health systems.

The two public health systems differ fundamentally according to their legal basis; in Denmark the broad Health Act includes all health system issues whereas in Slovakia the specific Public Health Act is quite independent of healthcare legislation. Key actors are easy to identify in Slovakia, mainly in the form of the public health authorities (national, regional), whereas they are distributed in Denmark amongst municipalities, regions, and the state. To compare the overall workforce is not possible without a detailed description of tasks and responsibilities. In financial terms, although there are large uncertainties related to the use of funding, about the same percentage of the budget of the respective Ministries (the Ministry of Health and Prevention in Denmark and the Ministry of Health in the Slovak Republic) was found for both countries. The core mission of key players is different; Danish municipalities have little health protection power compared to Slovak public health authorities. On the other hand, they have more opportunity to conduct disease prevention and health promotion activities.

Table 5.2 Public health systems of Denmark and the Slovak Republic

	Denmark	Slovak Republic
Key legislation	Health law (Sundhedsloven) from 16 June 2005, last version from 07 February 2008	Act on Protection, Support and Development of Public Health and on Amendments and Supplements to Certain Acts, No. 355/2007, last version from 19 May 2011
Key players	Regions: health care Municipalities: disease prevention and health promotion	Public Health Authority of the Slovak Republic Regional public health authorities
Centralization/ decentralization	Decentralized both in location of authorities and governance	Decentralized in location of authorities Centralized in governance
Estimated public health expenditure*	4,6% (2007), includes vaccination expenses (Disease Prevention Committee Report 2009)	2006–4.68% 2008–3.09% 2009–2.7% 2010–2.33% 2011–2.23%
Training	Three universities running BSc, MSc, and PhD programmes in public health	Six universities running BSc, MSc, and PhD programmes in public health
Core mission of key players	Health promotion, disease prevention and rehabilitation	Health protection, health promotion
Total health expenditure as % of GDP in 2007 (WHO HFA 2012)	9.7	7.7

*Estimated public health expenditures were calculated for both countries as percentage of total budget going to the health system from the national budget and targeted to public health/health promotion activities; for Denmark the national budget of 2007 was used.

In Slovakia, the Ministry of Health coordinates the cooperation of central governmental bodies in the sector of public health; it methodically regulates the performance of state health supervision, controls the performance of the public health system, and defines the directions of education in the field of the protection, promotion, and development of public health. The Public Health Authority of the Slovak Republic is the supreme office for the regional public health authorities; it manages, controls, and coordinates the execution of state administration carried out by them. According to the Slovak Act 355/2007, the Public Health Authority evaluates and approves HIA cases on a national level, and regional public health authorities on regional and local levels.

The national Public Health Authority is authorized to issue licenses to those who can conduct HIA or environmental health risk assessment. The proponent of any new proposal that is expected to have impact on health or may have health hazards is obliged to provide either an evaluation of health hazards or an HIA to the Public Health Authority or regional public health authorities who approve or reject the report.

Interestingly enough, in both countries, with apparently considerably different public health systems, the use of HIA became part of the agenda in early 2000.

Milestones in the implementation of HIA in Denmark and the Slovak Republic

First attempts to introduce HIA in Denmark can be traced back to 1996, when the Ministry of Health developed a proposal to the Danish government to introduce HIA on a national level. Unfortunately the government did not consider that proposal relevant (Bistrup and Kamper-Jørgensen 2005). The municipality of Nordborg, located in the South of Denmark, became a pioneer of HIA in the country by introducing HIA to all policy decisions by 2003. Other municipalities, some of them part of the Danish national or European network of WHO Healthy Cities, followed Nordborg to some extent by pushing the national level to develop a guidance document. The structural and administration reform introduced on 1 January 2007 delegated public health and health promotion responsibilities to municipalities (Andersen and Jensen 2010). This provided another important motivation for the national level to support implementation of HIA. A review of municipal health policies in spring 2008 disclosed that about 25–30% of municipalities aim to implement HIA within their routine work (Nikolajsen 2009). The National Board of Health responded by publication of a national guidance for the implementation of HIA in 2008 with a focus on the municipal level (Guliš et al. 2008). During spring 2009 there was an attempt initiated by the opposition parties in the Danish parliament to implement HIA by law on a national level, which failed. Recommendation No. 52 of the government established the Disease Prevention Committee, which in its final report (Disease Prevention Committee Report 2009) calls for HIA of policies on national and local levels when there is a potential for direct and relevant impact on the health of the population. Short-term training workshops on HIA were conducted in several municipalities between 2006 and 2010, partially supported by a European Commission (EC) funded project, 'Health impact assessment in new member states and accession countries—HIA-NMAC', which was coordinated by the

University of Southern Denmark. In 2009, Horsens municipality, a member of the Healthy City network, came up with an initiative to establish an informal group of municipalities who use HIA or work on its development. The network managed to get support from the National Board of Health for the development of systematic, likely e-learning based training modules and tool development for routine use of HIA. At present HIA is routinely used in several municipalities on both broader policies and projects.

In Slovakia, the first attempts to implement HIA came via EC- and WHO-funded project work. In the PHASE project conducted under the leadership of the WHO Healthy City network, two workshops were organized and a case study on HIA at the municipal level was conducted (Mannheimer et al. 2007). This was followed up by research work and another workshop conducted within the HIA-NMAC project together with WHO/Europe and Slovakia Biennial Collaborative Agreement (provided by the WHO Europe Rome office), this time on a national level with political representation and the support of the Ministry of Health in autumn 2006. Subsequently, five paragraphs on the implementation of HIA were included in newly adopted Act for the protection, promotion, and development of public health in 2007. However, enforcing the law for HIA was initially postponed from 2007 to January 2010 and then again until January 2011 as the final deadline. In 2008 the Chief Public Health Officer of the Slovak Republic initiated the establishment of a multi-sectoral expert group of 12: eight from the Public Health Authority and regional public health authorities and four from non-health sectors. This group has been assigned the task of taking the lead in the preparation of the public health system for full implementation of HIA by 1 January 2010, and organizing and conducting training sessions for other professionals. Information received at Slovak public health conferences on the first HIA licenses granted to experts and institutions in spring 2011 and the first HIA reports received by public health authorities in early summer 2011 demonstrate the success of this initiative. Another WHO Europe and Slovakia Biennial Collaborative Agreement workshop was set up in cooperation with the Ministry of Health of the Slovak Republic in February 2009. This workshop focused in particular on the social determinants of health and equity within HIA and formulated the following recommendations for action: conduct pilot HIA case studies, undertake further capacity-building on a regional level, and analyse the legislation from the point of view of mandatory EIAs with the inclusion of a health element. In autumn 2010 another workshop was conducted within the WHO Europe Biennial Collaborative Agreement, this time focusing specifically on the training of the eight experts, members of the multi-sectoral group, and tool development for HIA. The Public Health Authorities maintained the right to train, examine, and license potential professionally competent people as well as to evaluate and approve the HIA reports. At present, there are approximately 20 people who have already received a license, officially called a Certificate of Professional Competence, and can conduct HIA on a contractual basis.

Both cases sound like success stories on first examination. In the following section, we will analyse these cases from the point of view of implementation theory.

Implementation of HIA

The most influential definition of implementation is the one provided by Mazmanian and Sabatier (1983). Although to implement HIA could be considered as a policy decision, in fact it is a professional decision from the research level to policy and practice. HIA could be considered as an innovative work practice compared to traditional public health or standard impact assessment (IA) methods such as EIA, for example, therefore the diffusion of innovation (DoI) theory of Rogers (2003) suits the implementation of HIA. Rogers divides implementation into four key elements: innovation, social system, communication channels, and time. Time is further divided into stages of knowledge, persuasion, decision, implementation, and confirmation.

HIA is an innovation; IAs have been done for many years and EIA in particular has a long history, starting about the 1960s and being legislated first in the USA (National Environmental Policy Act 1969). Although health is to some extent part of an EIA, the focus is on environment and health is secondary; moreover, the role of the social determinants of health is often not considered in EIA. HIA is an innovation that focuses on health and applies research evidence from environmental, social, economic, and other areas into health. Apparently both Denmark and Slovakia accepted this and started to work on HIA implementation.

The social systems in the two countries differ quite substantially (see Table 5.1). Denmark has a long tradition of decentralized administration compared to Slovakia, which has, after being established in 1993, taken the first steps toward decentralization recently. The democratic parliamentary system-based governance is also older and more deeply established in Denmark. These parts of the social system are very important for the implementation of HIA because of the four key values of HIA described in the Gothenburg Consensus Paper (WHO 1999). Longer tradition favours Denmark in terms of the time of implementation and explains why Denmark started approximately 6 to 7 years earlier with attempts to implement HIA. The fourth key value of HIA—ethical use of evidence—and in fact the availability of evidence could be related to the existence of a wide public health infrastructure. This value seems to be more established in Slovakia where the network of public health authorities provides a robust knowledge and evidence base, and is has the necessary decision-making power. Denmark does not have that type of public health infrastructure available, so it relies more on academia and research than on local infrastructure. This fact explains to some extent why although Denmark started about 10 years earlier with implementation of HIA, at present the two countries are at about the same implementation level. To conclude, having a social system supporting all key values of HIA is an important enabler for implementation. Other important elements of the social system are in existence and the tradition of other IA techniques exists also; in Denmark it is the municipality who uses EIA, for example, so naturally it is easier to implement HIA at the same level whereas in Slovakia EIA is the responsibility of the Ministry of Environment so can be implemented at the national level.

Communication channels are important as they are expected to enhance the delivery of the message within the social system. In the case of HIA implementation, one needs to consider channels between research (where HIA was born), policy (where it becomes mandated), practice (where it is conducted), and training/education (where personal capacities are developed). Apparently in both Denmark and the Slovak Republic international organizations such as the EC and WHO provide major and important communication channels by bringing relevant players to conferences (for example Nordborg and the Healthy City movement), workshops (the HIA-NMAC and WHO Europe and Slovakia Biennial Collaborative Agreement workshops), and training events (a series of training workshops in Danish municipalities and the expert group in Slovakia). The most frequent communication channel in both cases is therefore the personal contact of researchers and educators with practitioners and policy makers at various levels (national, regional, and local).

Time is a very important element in the implementation process. The process starts with the existence of knowledge; this was reached around 1996 in Denmark and from 2003 to 2005 in the Slovak Republic. The persuasion phase needs to be considered together with the decision step. In the Danish case, initially persuasion was at the national level; this step is still not fully completed. At the local level, however, this phase ended in 2008/2009, when the national guidance document was published. Municipalities are gradually implementing HIA into routine practice and initiating new steps such as training possibilities and tool development. On the other hand, the Slovak Republic's persuasion phase has been completed and the decision was made by putting HIA into national law in 2007. Implementation of the law followed in January 2011, when the specific HIA paragraphs came into force. Both countries are in same position: the final phase of implementation with regard to time. They are conducting different levels of HIAs, developing new tools, testing new practices, looking for systematic capacity building, and so on, working on full achievement of HIA as an implemented working practice.

Hill and Hupe (2009) describe top-down and bottom-up approaches, or a synthesis (mix of both approaches), as possible directions for implementation. The Danish case started at the top level with the Ministry of Health initiative in 1996, which failed. First attempts in Slovakia were conducted at the municipal level, leading to a bottom-up direction. At present, these two cases show exactly the opposite directions; in Denmark success has been achieved by the bottom-up approach since the municipalities became the leaders, whereas in Slovakia HIA became a reality after several training events and modification of national legislation, thus demonstrating the top-down approach. Taking into account the political, historical, and public health systems of two countries, these results are unsurprising.

Conclusions

The double case study presented in this chapter offers relevant lessons with regard to the successful implementation of HIA in Denmark and Slovakia. The importance of the social system, time, and availability of capacities seem to be the most important factors in successful HIA implementation.

The role of the social system is not only about being supportive or unsupportive; it is more important to consider the perspective of finding the proper level of implementation (national versus local). Implementation usually starts with having knowledge of an innovation and that is located in the research or academic environment. Addressing the wrong level might seriously delay implementation of HIA, so researchers need to study the social system in depth before attempting to implement HIA. The answer to the question, whether implementation should be done using top-down or bottom-up approaches is revealed by the type of social system.

Time is a crucial and important variable; in both analysed cases it took many years to reach the current phase. Detailed knowledge of the social system and availability of personal capacities are the two key issues when examining how the timescale can be shortened.

In both countries a substantial amount of time was spent on the organization and conduct of training workshops and therefore on the development of personal capacities. This is a positive and necessary step; permanent systematic training is needed and effort has been made particularly in Denmark to reach that goal. However, having HIA and the determinants of health paradigm included in the regular public health curriculum would probably speed up the implementation process in both countries.

The comparison of the implementation processes within different contexts is always an interesting and promising task. In our Slovak case, the country can learn from the active and clearly health promotion-based approach to HIA implementation in Denmark. The process as described is fully in line with the definition of health promotion by the Ottawa Charter, especially the part of 'enabling people to increase control over and to improve their health' (WHO, 1986: 1). On the other hand, Slovakia has shown a quick and effective introduction of the personal competence licensing system, which is expected to contribute significantly to the quality of the process of HIA in the country. The regulatory approach employed in Slovakia is closely linked to the environmental health tradition of the country and its public health system.

In conclusion, and as a quest for further research following HIA practice in both countries (and probably in several others,) is needed, with the aim of identifying the real use of HIA recommendations, its achievements, and its impact on the policy-making processes, on project development, and, most importantly, on long-term improvements in population health.

Generic learning points

For public health practitioners and policy-makers

- Implementation of HIA should follow and respect the traditions of existing health and public health systems and cultures.
- Consultation with other countries that have already had some experience with HIA could enhance the implementation process.

For educators and researchers

- Academics should initiate inclusion of HIA into regular public health curricula (including lifelong learning of professionals). Moreover, elements of HIA should be included in the training of planners, policy-makers, and relevant stakeholders of sectors other than health.
- Research should focus on developing and testing standardized tools for screening, scoping, and risk appraisal.

References

Andersen, P.T. and Jensen, J.J. (2010) Health care reform in Denmark. *Scandinavian Journal of Public Health* 38: 246–252.

Bistrup, L.M. and Kamper-Jørgensen, F. (2005) *Sundhedskonsekvensvurderinger; Koncept. Perspektiver. Anvendelse i stat, amter og kommuner.* [Health impact assessment;

concept, perspectives, use in national, regional and local level.] Copenhagen: Statens Institute for Folkesundhed.

Disease Prevention Committee Report (2009) *Vi kan leve laengere og sundere, Forebyggesleskommisionenrapport.* Copenhagen: Forebyggelseskommision. Available at <http://www.forebyggelseskommissionen.dk/Files/Billeder/betaenkning/ Forebyggelseskommissionen__rapport.pdf>. Accessed 13 July 2011.

Eurostat (2011) Country profiles. Available at <http://epp.eurostat.ec.europa.eu/guip/ introAction.do?profile=cpro&theme=eurind&lang=en>. Accessed June 2011.

Gothenburg Consensus Paper (1999) *Health Impact Assessment: main concepts and suggested approach.*, Brussels: WHO European Centre for Health Policy. Available at <http://www.apho.org.uk/resource/item.aspx?RID=44163>. Accessed 14 February 2012.

Guliš, G., Gry, P., and Kræmer, S.R.J. (2008) *Sundhedskonsekvensvurdering—fra teori til praksis.* [Health impact assessment—from theory to practice.], Copenhagen: National Board of Health (Sundhedstyrelsen).

Health Statistics Yearbook of Slovak Republic (2007) National Health Information Centre of the Slovak Republic. Available at <http://www.nczisk.sk/Documents/rocenky/ rocenka_2007.pdf>. Accessed 14 February 2012.

Hill, M. and Hupe, P. (2009) *Implementing Public Policy,* 2nd edition. London: Sage Publications.

Mannheimer, L.N ., Guliš, G., Lehto, J., and Ostlin, P. (2007) Introducing health impact assessment: an analysis of political and administrative intersectoral working methods. *European Journal of Public Health* 17 (5): 526–553.

Mazmanian, D.A. and Sabatier, P.A. (1983) *Implementation and public policy.* Lexington, KY: Lexington Books.

National Environmental Policy Act (1969) Available at <http://ceq.hss.doe.gov/nepa/regs/ nepa/nepaeqia.htm>.

Nikolajsen, L.T. (2009) *Implementering af sundhedskonsekvensvuredring.* [Implementation of health impact assessment]. Masters thesis. Esbjerg: University of Southern Denmark.

Rogers, E.M. (2003) *Diffusion of Innovations,* 5th edition. New York: Free Press, a division of Simon & Schuster, Inc.

WHO (1986) Ottawa Charter for health promotion. Available at <http://www.who.int/ healthpromotion/conferences/previous/ottawa/en/>. Accessed 12 August 2011.

WHO-HFA (2012) European Health for All database. Available at <http://data.euro.who. int/hfadb/>. Accessed on 14 February 2012.

Chapter 6

The Ruhr metropolitan area in Germany: rapid health impact assessment of novel spatial planning

Rainer Fehr

Introduction

As underlined by authoritative sources (for example, the Commission on Social Determinants of Health 2008), spatial planning offers unique gateways to health protection and promotion. Compared to the opportunities, current practice lags behind. This chapter outlines a specific planning process and describes the input originating from a rapid health impact assessment (HIA) as well as the reactions received from the planning authorities. It goes on to investigate how to strengthen the position of the health sector for improving the consideration of health in such situations.

This chapter endorses a comprehensive and integrative approach to HIA, based on human ecology, to adequately consider 'human health' as a subject of societal efforts of protection and promotion.

Background

Population health is known to be influenced by activities in multiple societal sectors. Public planning aims to accommodate a range of societal goals (Fürst 2008). In this context, impact assessments (IAs), for example strategic environmental assessment (SEA), play a key role (Scholles 2008). The involvement of health professionals in planning is geared towards harvesting the opportunities and optimizing the health impacts of planning decisions, including spatial planning. In many regions, including the state of North Rhine-Westphalia (*Nordrhein-Westfalen*, NRW), this is also required by public health law (*Gesetz über den öffentlichen Gesundheitsdienst des Landes Nordrhein-Westfalen*; ÖGDG NRW 1997).

With approximately 18 million inhabitants, NRW is the most populous federal state of Germany. More than 25% of the state population live in the metropolitan region called the Ruhr area (*Ruhrgebiet*)—the 'German megacity' and the place of residence for 5 million inhabitants. Many of the Ruhr area cities previously were centres of heavy industry, and they are now undergoing conversion.

Not surprisingly, spatial planning in the Ruhr area poses considerable challenges. There are several planning processes here, intertwined with one another. One example is the 'Concept Ruhr' initiative, involving more than 40 cities/communities and three counties, which focuses on economic development (Wirtschaftsförderung metropoleruhr 2011).

Around the turn of the millennium, in a research and development project entitled City 2030 (*Stadt 2030*), the Technical University of Dortmund coordinated a project called Region of Ruhr Cities 2030 (*Städteregion Ruhr 2030*), featuring the motto 'Cooperation and Self-Will' (*Kooperation und Eigensinn*). Based on this project, the network Region of Ruhr cities 2030 (*Städteregion Ruhr 2030*) was formed, which today comprises 11 cities (Städteregion Ruhr 2030 2011a). Activities include a Master plan Ruhr (Städteregion Ruhr 2030 2011b), a coordinated monitoring activity of the housing market (*Regionale Wohnungsmarktbeobachtung*), a joint initiative Ruhr valley (*Gemeinschaftsinitiative Ruhrtal*), and other related activities.

In the beginning, the project required the participating cities to contractually agree to coordinate their spatial planning. In 2003, a city–regional contract (*Stadtregionaler Kontrakt*) was negotiated and enacted. In this contract, a joint Regional Land Use Plan (*Regionaler Flächennutzungsplan*, RFNP) was listed as a key project (Städteregion Ruhr 2030 2011c). This novel approach of joint spatial planning is the topic of the case study described in this chapter.

Case study

Policy being examined

As mentioned, in 2005 six cities of the Ruhr area established a planning consortium (*Planungsgemeinschaft*) in order to prepare a joint RFNP. The consortium members were the cities of Bochum, Essen, Gelsenkirchen, Herne, Muelheim/Ruhr, and Oberhausen. The population of these cities in 2005 was 1.8 million (area = 680 km², population density = 2664 per km²). The cities represent a core area of the Ruhrgebiet.

The RFNP is unique because it combines the function of a regional plan (*Regionalplan*) and a joint local spatial plan (*gemeinsamer Flächennutzungsplan*). This type of plan had been introduced in 2004 to state planning legislation. In 2006, a concomitant committee (*Verfahrensbegleitender Ausschuss*) was formed to facilitate regional coordination. In 2007, the formal planning procedure started. Several steering bodies were involved: one consisting of chief officers (*Amtsleiter*), one of heads of planning departments (*Bau- und Planungsdezernenten*), one project group for RFNP, and one for environment.

In 2007, there was early public and stakeholder participation. In addition to legal requirements and the state planning framework, a range of technical specialist documents (*Fachbeiträge*) was utilized in preparing the RFNP, including ones on nature conservancy, soil protection, water management, agriculture, forests, regional climate, industry, crafts, and trade.

There were two waves of public and stakeholder involvement (*Öffentlichkeits- und Trägerbeteiligung*). The 'early' involvement from November 2007 until February 2008 included 19 public meetings, spawning approximately 6000 suggestions for change. Also, 256 agencies and institutions, including those dedicated to public interest (*Träger öffentlicher Belange, TÖB*), were involved, producing 115 statements with approximately 590 suggestions. Secondly, there was 'formal' involvement of stakeholders and the public, in the period October to December 2008. This included public display (*Auslegung*) and debate (*Erörterung*) of the draft RFNP, the Environmental Report, and the responses received so far.

In the draft version, the spatial plan consisted of 45 different items, including maps and texts. The planning policy was subject to SEA, necessitating an environmental report (*Umweltbericht*) accompanied by additional maps (Box 6.1).

After the two waves of public and stakeholder involvement, in the period from May to June 2009 the city councils of the six RFNP cities resolved to approve the RFNP (now consisting of 43 items) and submitted it to the NRW Ministry of Economics, Small- and Medium-sized Businesses, and Energy for approval (*Genehmigung*). The ministry then defined some constraints, necessitating another round of cities' resolutions. Finally, the RFNP was officially published. It was the first such plan in Germany, and came into force on 3 May 2010.

The RFNP replaced existing land utilization plans and sections of the regional development plans. Incidentally, the NRW State Planning Act (*Landesplanungsgesetz*) of 2010 does not provide the option of RFNP. Instead, there will be a regional plan for a larger area. For the interim period, the planning consortium is authorized to update the RFNP.

Box 6.1 Materials reflecting the RFNP draft plan of 2008

◆ Proposed resolution (*Beschlussvorlage*)

◆ Map (*Plankarte*)

◆ Rationale (*Begründung*) with 10 additional maps (*Erläuterungskarten*)

◆ Environmental report (*Umweltbericht*)—required by SEA—with 12 thematic maps (*Themenkarten*)

◆ Seven summaries of characteristics (*Steckbriefe*)

◆ Several further summaries, listings, overviews, and synopses

Rapid HIA of the novel RFNP

In this comprehensive RFNP planning process, LIGA.NRW was asked to act as the 'institution responsible for public concerns' (*Träger öffentlicher Belange*) and to support the coverage of health aspects in this policy procedure. (LIGA.NRW was the Institute of Health and Work North Rhine-Westphalia. Since 1 January 2012 it has been transformed into the NRW Center for Health, <http://www.lzg.gc.nrw.de.>). This was done by providing a rapid health impact assessment, based primarily on the 45 items of the draft RFNP (Fehr and Welteke 2008; Volmer et al. 2010).

For this situation, it was decided to focus on the following aspects:

◆ evaluation of health-related topics already touched upon in the planning process so far
◆ where appropriate, pinpoint additional topics, indicating both health risks and opportunities associated with the RFNP
◆ suggest ways to gain a fuller coverage of health, beyond what was possible in this 'rapid' assessment.

It was decided to apply the following methods: document analysis, process participation, and expert judgement. The planning materials were examined in detail and assessed from the background of international experiences with planning involvement and HIA at large. It was found that the environmental report in particular, prepared as part of the pertinent SEA, contained comprehensive descriptions, assessments, and map-based visualizations concerning human health. This was related to both the status quo and the impacts of future designations of residential areas, commercial areas, and transport infrastructure.

In summary, the environmental report discussed a range of different health issues, including mortality, life expectancy, hospitalization, land use, soil pollution, brownfields, ground-, surface, and drinking water, floods, air pollution (including particulate matter), NOx, local climate, disaster prevention and response (Seveso II-Council Directive, 1996), noise and vibrations, especially from highways, railways, industry, light pollution, offensive odours, electro-magnetic fields, waste disposal, recreation, and leisure activities.

To some extent, the rapid HIA evolved as a response to how health topics were handled in the set of RFNP documents. Other parts of the HIA report refer to additional substantive and procedural issues, including a set of recommendations from a population health perspective. The structure of the HIA statement is shown in Box 6.2.

Suggestions were made about how to integrate suggested changes into the existing documents. The substantive issues raised included population health status, physical activity, gender issues, and diversity. As for population health status, it was stated that existing health statistics and local health reports should be integrated into the RFNP procedure, especially for describing the status quo of population health, for identifying areas of particular concern, potentially for deriving health targets, and for developing specific improvement strategies. Taking it further, it was suggested that the concept of burden of disease including prevention potentials, be applied and to relate it to opportunities arising from the RFNP.

An example of such opportunity refers to physical activity. The RFNP was seen as an occasion to significantly increase the spatial requirements and facilitating factors for physical activity. As a third area of substantive topics, the rapid HIA addressed gender issues, high-risk groups, and disabled persons. The spatial plan was seen as an occasion to promote social inclusion, thus fostering health-related equity.

Box 6.2 Structure of LIGA.NRW's rapid HIA report

Title: Expert statement concerning the draft of RFNP City region Ruhr (*Stellungnahme zum Vorentwurf des RFNP Städteregion Ruhr*), January 2008

Report structure

1. Planning region and health situation

2. Impacts of the planning project on population health determinants, as found in the environmental report, including noise, mortality, and morbidity, expertise on human health, environmental impacts of low-/ high-frequency electro-magnetic fields

3. Concise summaries of characteristics (*Steckbriefe*) concerning specific areas

4. Additional explanations concerning topics with special significance for health, which should be elaborated on in the emerging RFNP

    4.1 Physical immobility and planning—preventive strategies to pro-mote physical mobility in the spatial planning context

    4.2 Gender issues and diversity

Appendix: Text elements suggested to complement the rationale of the RFNP, concerning (i) housing and (ii) the economy.

Concerning amendments to the body of RFNP documents, LIGA.NRW suggested that in order to underline the relevance of health for regional development and in analogy to other topics, a section on human health should be included in the planning document, and a separate report or technical paper on this issue should be prepared. Concerning the environmental report, it was pointed out that existing text passages on environmental risks and resources (including noise, recreation, green spaces, and so on) needed to be interpreted much more explicitly with respect to their health implications, i.e. changes of the burden of disease. In order to strengthen the weight of health concerns for fair balancing, the concise summaries of characteristics (*Steckbriefe*) would need to include health considerations more extensively.

Finally, several procedural issues were raised, for example a need to balance different targets and values (including health), legal requirements to be fully exploited, and health issues to be given more weight than they received in the past.

As mentioned above, numerous agencies and institutions were involved in the process. From the planners' perspective, LIGA.NRW was merely one of more than 250 such institutions, alongside private enterprises including energy providers, various agencies (especially from transport sector), religious groups (Catholic, Protestant, Jewish), chamber of architects, association of architects, universities, and sports clubs.

The rapid HIA was regarded by the planning officials as one of the 115 statements received altogether, and the HIA report was seen as representing 14 different specific suggestions (from a total of 590 suggestions received). As part of the RFNP planning process, planning officials explicitly responded to the suggestions received. Concerning the rapid HIA, the suggestions identified by the planning officials as well as their responses are shown in Table 6.1.

The responses to HIA-related suggestions can be summarized as follows. Six (out of 14) suggestions were turned down, for a variety of reasons. One suggestion was merely declared

Table 6.1 Rapid HIA: suggestions identified by planning officials and the official responses

	Category	Suggestion (headline) in rapid HIA	Reaction from planning officials
1.	Miscellaneous	Additional text on health, if possible a whole section dedicated to health	Suggestion not accepted
2.	Miscellaneous	Gender issues and diversity a) More attention should be given to diversity	Suggestion partially accepted
		b) Gender mainstreaming should be heeded	Statements taken notice of
3.	Miscellaneous	Give special attention to the promotion of physical exercise within spatial planning	Suggestion not accepted
4.	Housing	Additional text on 'healthy housing'	Suggestion is already accepted
5.	Economy	Add text on the societal role of health and health economy	Suggestion partially accepted
6.	Environmental assessment	The environmental report needs to be more precise concerning the influence on health determinants and on human health, including interactions	Suggestion accepted to a large extent
7.	Environmental assessment	Intensive usage of existing data, information, and reports on regional mortality and morbidity	Suggestion not accepted
8.	Environmental assessment	Technical paper dedicated to human health	Suggestion not accepted
9.	Environmental assessment	In the environmental report, the coverage of humans/human health needs to be extended and specified	Suggestion accepted
10.	Environmental assessment	Final treatment and interpretation of the partial results concerning the Seveso II directive	Statement taken notice of The safety areas and safety distances will be accounted for in the environmental assessment

(continued)

Table 6.1 (*Continued*)

	Category	Suggestion (headline) in rapid HIA	Reaction from planning officials
11.	Environmental assessment	Need to ensure that the contents of the 'Summaries of characteristics' are heeded in future planning steps	Suggestion not accepted
12.	Environmental assessment	Identify foreseeable noise conflicts and earmark for conflict resolution in next planning phase	Statement is taken notice of
13.	Environmental assessment	In the environmental report, the role of environmental resources (including open space) needs to be discussed in more detail	Suggestion accepted (to some extent)
14.	Environmental assessment	Add information on low-/ high-frequency radiation	Suggestion not accepted

'taken notice of', four suggestions were accepted partially, and three were accepted without (major) qualification, with one of them seen as 'already accepted'.

In summary, this rapid HIA was embedded in a novel joint planning process on a regional level. The results were directly used to inform the planning and policy procedure, with a limited but noticeable influence on the regional plan.

Conclusions

From the experiences gained in this rapid HIA (and other HIAs), the following can be concluded. Spatial planning offers a variety of opportunities to promote and protect human health. In a country with no explicit HIA programme, it is technically possible to contribute, from a health perspective, to a regional planning process. The planning procedures—especially in a densely populated area—involve large numbers of institutions and comprehensive public involvement. In such a situation, the number of statements and suggestions received by planning officials can be substantial, making the HIA contribution just one out of many.

For those testifying for health it is a challenge to adequately understand the ramifications of the planning process and to adequately cover the health issues at stake, especially in the absence of standard procedures and tools. For those managing the planning process, it is likewise challenging to evaluate and integrate the multitude of suggestions received. Even if the overall response to the HIA is not unfavourable, the success can turn out to be limited, from a public health perspective, and may seem to be not commensurate with the weight that the topic would deserve.

In our experience, the situation described here is not a singularity but rather a 'typical' case, therefore structural changes and adjustments appear necessary. The HIA exercise reported here was instrumental in establishing the need for strengthening 'health' and the health sector in inter-sectoral cooperation. From this and other HIA examples, we concluded that there is a need to strengthen the position of the health sector and to streamline health-related contributions to planning processes. Current efforts to do so include: (i) establishing closer connections between HIA and other governance tools, including health targets, health reporting, health conferences, and health awards, (ii) preparing departmental health plans (*Fachpläne Gesundheit*), in analogy to other sectoral plans on local and regional level, e.g. housing plan, sports plan, educational plan, and (iii) better understanding of the commonalities, differences, and interrelationships of various types of IA (e.g. in the environmental arena), and promotion of closer cooperation among them.

Generic learning points

For public health practitioners and policy-makers

- Opportunities worth being used: HIA, for example as it is applied to spatial planning, offers significant entry points to promote and protect human health. These opportunities can constitute a key element of regional and local health policy development. They deserve to be used systematically.

- Utilization gap: In Germany, and apparently in many other countries, the health opportunities offered by HIA are under-used. This 'utilization gap' is not entirely surprising. As illustrated above, planning is a complex procedure, involving large numbers of stakeholders and comprehensive discussions.

- Growing agreement to 'close the gap': There is growing consensus among planners and health professionals to close this gap. Spatial planning could evolve into a major, and universally accepted, approach to health protection and promotion, and a key component of professional toolkits. Partially related to the experience described in this chapter, health experts together with planners and environmental impact assessors in Germany now continuously cooperate in a working group and prepare guidelines.

- Flexibility: HIA needs to be seen as a *flexible* tool—situations for applying HIA differ considerably, so the tool has to be adjusted. The basic HIA idea is straightforward. The adaptations require creativity and endurance but are feasible and potentially rewarding.

- Supporting activities: In the inter-sector debate in Germany, numerous sectors support their case with specific departmental plans (*Fachpläne*), e.g. on housing, sports, or nature conservancy. Current efforts to establish such plans for the health sector can contribute to strengthening HIA.

For educators and researchers

- As illustrated by the case presented here, HIA takes place at the intersection of different 'cultures', especially (health) science on one side and (e.g. regional) planning on the other. Planners often receive large numbers of suggestions. In this situation, successful interdisciplinary communication is crucial, therefore interdisciplinary communication in HIA contexts should be introduced to the curricula of both public health and planning professionals.

- Beyond communication, curricula for planners should provide a basic understanding of physical and social health determinants as well as of health-related impact assessments.

- For public health professionals, both the HIA 'vision' and the specific methodologies need to be taught, practiced, critically discussed, and integrated into the professional toolkit, alongside other types of advanced health assessments.

References

Commission on Social Determinants of Health (2008) *Closing the gap in a generation: Health equity through action on the social determinants of health.* Final report. Geneva: WHO. Available at <http://www.who.int/social_determinants/thecommission/final-report/en/index.html>. Accessed 29 December 2011.

European Commission (1996) Council Directive (1996) *96/82/EC on the control of major-accident hazards involving dangerous substances.* Brussels: European Commission. Brussels

Fehr, R. and Welteke, R. (2008) Joint regional land utilization plan (Regionaler Flächennutzungsplan, RFNP) of Ruhr area cities: Rapid health impact assessment. *Umweltmed Forsch Prax* 13 (5): 274.

Fürst, D. (2008) Begriff der Planung und Entwicklung der Planung in Deutschland, in Fürst, D., and Scholles, F. (eds), *Handbuch Theorien und Methoden der Raum- und Umweltplanung*, 3rd edition. Dortmund: Verlag Dorothea Rohn, pp 21–47 (Ch. 2.1).

ÖGDG NRW (1997) §8 Mitwirkung an Planung, Vom 25 November. Available at <https://recht.nrw.de/lmi/owa/br_bes_text?print=1&anw_nr=2&gld_nr=2&ugl_nr=2120&val=4659&ver=0&sg=&menu=1&aufgehoben=N&keyword=ögdg&bes_id=4659>. Accessed 29 December 2011.

Scholles, F. (2008) Entwicklungsplanungen versus Folgenprüfungen—Verfahren und Planungsmethoden, in Fürst, D. and Scholles, F. (eds), *Handbuch Theorien und*

Methoden der Raum- und Umweltplanung, 3rd edition. Dortmund: Verlag Dorothea Rohn, pp 245–264 (Ch. 3.2).

Städteregion Ruhr 2030 (2011a) Städteregion Ruhr. Available at <http://www.staedteregion-ruhr-2030.de>. Accessed 29 December 2011.

Städteregion Ruhr 2030 (2011b) Master plan Ruhr. Available at <http://www.staedteregion-ruhr-2030.de/cms/masterplan_ruhr.html>. Accessed 29 December 2011.

Städteregion Ruhr 2030 (2011c) Regionaler Flächennutzungsplan. Available at <http://www.staedteregion-ruhr-2030.de/cms/regionaler_flaechennutzungsplan.html>. Accessed 29 December 2011.

Volmer, M., Welteke, R., and Fehr, R. (2010) *Berücksichtigung des Schutzgutes 'Menschliche Gesundheit' im Rahmen der Aufstellung des 'Regionalen Flächennutzungsplans der Planungsgemeinschaft Städteregion Ruhr'*. UVP report 1+2 2010, pp 54–60. Hamm: UVP-Gesellschaft.

Wirtschaftsförderung metropoleruhr (2011) Konzept Ruhr. Available at <http://www.konzept-ruhr.de>. Accessed 29 December 2011.

Chapter 7

Health impact assessment and its role in shaping government policy-making: the use of health impact assessment at national policy level in England

Salim Vohra, Gifty Amo-Danso,
and Judith Ball

Introduction

England has been at the forefront of health impact assessment (HIA) theory and practice since its inception in the early 1980s. Project-level HIA is now widely undertaken in England on housing, regeneration, waste, energy, and transport projects (see HIA Gateway, <www.hiagateway.org.uk>). Policy-level HIA is less widespread, with HIAs of London's key strategies and some other regional-level spatial and transport strategies being notable examples. It is unclear why there is this difference in practice between project- and policy-level HIAs. Two reasons identified by the UK Council for Science and Technology in its 2006 review were the limited ability of policy-makers outside the Department of Health (DH) to identify the public health evidence and advice they required, and the limited ability of DH policy-makers to influence other departments on the health impacts of their policies (Council for Science and Technology 2006). Other reasons for this may be the more established use of environmental impact assessment (EIA) to assess projects, making it easier to commission and conduct HIA at project level, the mimicking of the steps in the EIA process and its methodology in project-level HIA, and the loss of the Health Development Agency, which was subsumed into the National Institute of Clinical Excellence (NICE), which had, between 1999 and 2005, acted as a key driver for HIA use locally and nationally (NICE 2009).

England is unusual internationally in that an impact assessment (IA) is mandatory for all new national policies and taking account of health is an embedded part of the IA process (HM Government 2011a). Given the ongoing international debate about if, and how, HIA should be integrated into the policy process, England provides an interesting case study of the opportunities and challenges of incorporating HIA into the national policy development process. This chapter outlines how the IA process works in England and how HIA is embedded within the government IA process, and includes findings from an evaluation into how HIA was used by Government Departments between 2007 and 2009, and a discussion of the barriers and facilitating factors to the use of HIA in government policy-making.

The IA process in England

In England, the IA process is intended to be a continuous process and tool that helps policy-makers (civil servants and politicians) to 'think through the reasons for government intervention, to weigh up various options for achieving an objective and to understand the consequences of a proposed intervention' (HM Government 2011b: 4). This includes assessing its likely monetary costs and benefits, and the risks that might impact on public, private, or civil society organizations, including any additional regulatory burdens. In England, all governments since the 1980s have seen new legislation as an additional requirement and burden on society, particularly business, which can hinder entrepreneurship and enterprise, and in turn economic growth and development, as well as new ways of delivering public services. The IA process has been developed from the HM Treasury Department's policy appraisal guidance, popularly titled 'The Green Book' (HM Treasury 2011).

IAs are typically carried out by a government department's economic analysts and policy leads, who are civil servants (public officials). In some cases, external consultants are commissioned to conduct an IA or parts of an IA. Completed IAs, on a range of policy options or a preferred option, are published in draft form for consultation before being finalized. This is generally done through the websites of both the government department sponsoring the policy and the department that oversees the IA process (formerly the Department for Business, Enterprise and Regulatory Reform, now the Department for Business, Innovation and Skills, DBIS).

Historically, in England, policy assessment of national policy started with 'compliance cost assessments' in 1985, which became 'risk assessments' in 1996, 'regulatory impact assessments' in 1998 and 'impact assessments' in 2007 (Cabinet Office & Better Regulation Executive 2006). In 2011, further changes were made to the IA guidance, toolkit, and template (HM Government 2011a–d). The two key drivers for changing the policy IA process have been the twin political objectives of reducing the regulatory burden on business and improving the effectiveness and efficiency of policy-making. Although there have been differences in the format in which IAs are presented to government over the last 10 years, there are, and have been, strong similarities and consistencies in the aims, objectives, and process of IA.

The place of HIA within the IA process in England

The DH is England's national agency for health, with both policy and operational functions. This is the same as the national Ministry of Health found in other countries internationally. DH has been the champion for health and wellbeing impacts to be routinely considered within the IA and policy development process. It therefore takes responsibility for providing guidance on how to consider health and wellbeing impacts, and how to undertake HIA as part of the IA process to other government departments.

DH produced one of the earliest national documents on policy HIA, *Policy Appraisal and Health*, first published in 1996 and updated in 2004 (Department of Health 2004). The document is a guide to applying the general IA process and The Green Book guidance in relation to the health and wellbeing impacts of new policies. DH has been involved in the evolution of the overall IA process and the way health and wellbeing impacts are considered across government since that time. The importance of ensuring health and wellbeing is maintained and enhanced rose up the policy agenda in the 1990s and has been explicitly mentioned in England's national health strategies since that time (Wismar et al. 2007).

The 2011 HIA guidance is made up of five stages (Department of Health 2010a–d):

1. screening (whether or not to do an HIA)
2. identifying health impacts
3. prioritizing health impacts
4. quantifying or describing impacts
5. providing recommendations to enable the greatest health gains to be achieved.

Where policy development and IA teams consider health and wellbeing may be affected by a new policy they must undertake the screening stage of the HIA process. This involves answering five questions. If all five questions are answered 'no' then HIA does not need to be undertaken. If any of the questions result in a 'yes', then Stages 2 to 3 are completed. If Stage 3 does not identify any 'important' health impacts then the HIA can be considered complete at this stage. If there are important impacts then Stages 4 and 5 are completed.

Important impacts are considered to be those that may:

◆ impact on the whole population or on specific age groups, ethnic groups, religious groups, or socioeconomic groups

◆ be difficult to remedy or have an irreversible impact

◆ be medium to long term

◆ cause a great deal of public concern or

◆ have cumulative or synergistic impacts.

The guidance recommends that a multi-disciplinary IA team that is headed by a policy lead and made up of analysts, economists, social researchers, and subject matter specialists, conducts the HIA. The findings of the HIA are then integrated into the overall economic analysis and policy options discussion within the overall IA.

How health, wellbeing, and HIA are considered by English government departments

In 2009/2010 the authors evaluated the use of HIA and how health and wellbeing were considered within England's IA process. Not all the findings of the evaluation are in the public domain and this chapter only has space to discuss the key public findings. Additional information can be found in the summary report *Putting Health in the Policy Picture* (Department of Health and Institute of Occupational Medicine 2010). The IOM Centre for Health Impact Assessment at the Institute of Occupational Medicine has conducted additional independent follow-up work since 2011 (Vohra et al. 2011).

The authors reviewed all the IAs published from November 2007 (when the previous guidance was introduced) to March 2009. We also had informal discussions with analysts from some government departments to gain further insight into departmental attitudes, opinions, and practices in relation to HIA.

We found a lot of variation in how health and wellbeing were considered and assessed both within, as well as across, government departments. While many policy and IA teams did consider the health and wellbeing impacts of new policies, few considered these impacts systematically and comprehensively or by conducting an HIA. The full range of social determinants of health was rarely, if ever, identified, and there was little, or no, focus on health inequalities, health equity, or the distribution of health and wellbeing impacts. Inequalities issues were only explicitly considered when they were already on the political agenda, e.g. fuel poverty and equality of opportunity and access. What little discussion of health and wellbeing impacts we found was generally policy-relevant and appropriate. Health and wellbeing issues were often seen as social welfare and quality of life issues. That is, while a range of what could be called public health issues were clearly on the policy agenda, policy and IA teams were not necessarily using a health lens to identify and analyse these (see Table 7.1).

Table 7.1 Examples of health and wellbeing impacts considered but often seen as social welfare and quality of life issues in IAs in 2007–2009

Policy area	Health and wellbeing impacts routinely considered
Crime reduction	Reduced healthcare costs to victims and the National Health Service (NHS)
	Increased healthcare costs associated with imprisonment for both offenders and their families
	Global health effects of reduced organized crime, e.g. drug use and smuggling, people trafficking, and commercial sex work.
	Victims of white collar crime, e.g. stress and loss of life savings
Alcohol	Cost to the NHS
	Cost to victims of alcohol-related crime
	Costs of policing alcohol-related safety issues
Terrorism	Chronic stress due to worry and fear
	Physical and mental health impacts of a catastrophic terrorist act
Apprenticeships	Wellbeing impact of increased skills and wages
	Equity impact of access to apprenticeships for women, the disabled, and minority groups
Formal and informal learning	Enhanced uptake of health promotion messages, improved mental wellbeing
	Better job opportunities, reduced unemployment
	Poor health/disability a barrier to learning
Climate change	Fuel poverty
	Outdoor air quality
	Indoor air quality and ventilation
	Excess deaths associated with heat waves
	Death/injury due to flooding
Housing/ regeneration	Decent homes
	Overcrowding
	Security
	Enabling people to staying in their existing homes
Fire service	Fire safety

(continued)

Table 7.1 (*Continued*)

Policy area	Health and wellbeing impacts routinely considered
Environmental protection	Air quality Noise Biodiversity
Aviation	Air quality Noise
Public TRANSPORT	Access to services Inequity in access to transport
Dangerous Goods	Safety, in particular exposure to toxins
Road networks	Traffic safety Noise Physical activity
Driver licensing	Traffic safety

Reproduced from Vohra, S., Amo-Danso, G., and Ball, J., Further research on how health is considered in England's national policymaking, IOM Centre for Health Impact Assessment, Institute of Occupational Medicine (unpublished). Copyright © 2011, with permission from the author.

Few IAs quantified the potential health and wellbeing impacts in ways that could be incorporated into the core economic analysis. Where health and wellbeing impacts were quantified and monetized as costs and benefits this was generally because there were established and accepted departmental or cross-departmental methods for quantifying and monetizing the impacts, e.g. quality-adjusted life years, cost of victim harm, cost of substance misuse, air pollution mortality and morbidity costs, and value of a life saved/fatality prevented.

There was very low awareness and use of DH's HIA guidance. There was also little explicit use of public health evidence to justify judgements on the potential health and wellbeing impacts. In only a few cases were DH involved in supporting the analysis of health impacts, e.g. alcohol and air-quality strategies.

IA was often seen as a check to ensure that there were no unintended negative impacts of the policy. This was evidenced by a number of IAs stating that '... there are no detrimental health impacts arising from these proposals... ' or words to that effect. Positive health impacts were seen as requiring little or no analysis. Where positive health and wellbeing impacts were considered briefly they tended to be those that were high on the policy agenda, for example physical activity in relation to green space and sustainable transport policies.

Influence and value of HIA in the IA and policy process in England

We found that health and wellbeing can be an important driver in the policy development process where there is media and public interest, advocacy from DH, alignment of the departmental agenda with health and wellbeing, and the ability to quantify and monetize health and wellbeing impacts in a credible way that moves the issue up the policy agenda or builds a better case for the need for policy. Examples of policies where health and wellbeing acted as a driver include alcohol, environmental tobacco smoke, human trafficking, commercial sex work, and education policies.

However, HIA and the consideration of health and wellbeing impacts have little or no influence, and tend not to be done, where:

◆ policies are seen to be positive or neutral in terms of their health and wellbeing impacts

◆ similarly, policy options with politically or departmentally significant negative health and wellbeing impacts are screened out at an early stage of the policy development process (because it is assumed that no important negative impacts are present in the remaining options) or

◆ IAs are seen to be a 'rubber stamping' exercise because decisions have already been made at the political level to go in a certain policy direction.

Our work to date strongly suggests that HIAs have the potential to add value to the national IA and policy development processes by:

◆ helping to keep citizens—rather than just private, public, and third sector organizations—at the centre of policymaking

◆ providing a better and more complete documentation of positive and negative health and wellbeing impacts to ensure that policies take full account of public interests, and the full costs and benefits are explicitly weighed up

◆ bringing attention to the distribution of impacts and thereby alerting policy-makers to policy options that are likely to widen or narrow the gap between privileged and vulnerable groups

◆ helping to develop mitigation and enhancement measures that improve the implementation and outcomes of a policy

◆ helping to better frame the problem by providing baseline health and wellbeing information and analysis to increase the weight and priority given to a particular policy or policy option

◆ supporting the achievement of a government department's objectives, especially those that are cross-cutting, by identifying the direct and indirect health and wellbeing benefits of a policy and thereby strengthening the case for a proposed policy and justifying public spending priorities

♦ helping to influence how similar policies are developed in the future by providing an example of, and approach to, fully considering the potential health and wellbeing impacts of such policies.

Barriers and facilitating factors to the use of HIA in government policy-making

Our experience and research suggests that the key barriers to the use of HIA in policy-making are:

♦ limited time and resources where HIA is seen as a 'nice to do' extra

♦ health and wellbeing being seen as secondary and not explicitly aligned to a government department's objectives

♦ low awareness of the full range of public health and wellbeing impacts that can result from a policy

♦ low awareness of the HIA guidance and expertise that is available

♦ lack of scrutiny of how appropriately health and wellbeing impacts are considered in IAs and the lack of enforcement of the obligation to conduct an HIA when relevant

♦ lack of HIA and 'healthy public policy' focused public health expertise at national policy level

♦ lack of high-quality, policy-relevant and accessible public health evidence in many policy areas

♦ methodological challenges to quantifying and monetizing health and wellbeing impacts in many policy areas.

Key facilitating factors to the use of HIA are:

♦ having explicit government department objectives on the protection and promotion of public health and/or the natural and built environment

♦ mutual interest among governmental departments in achieving jointly agreed or aligned departmental and whole of government objectives

♦ health and wellbeing issues with a clear and policy-relevant evidence base that can support the case for new policy.

Conclusions

The authors are not aware of any other evaluation of the use of HIA and how health and wellbeing are considered during the development of national policies. The findings of our work are broadly supported by other research on policy level HIAs and the use of HIA to support the health in all policies (HiAP) agenda (Government of Quebec 2008; Cole and Fielding 2008; Public Health Advisory Committee 2007; Kemm 2006; Mahoney and Durham 2002; Varela Put et al. 2001). HIA is one important way of achieving HiAP but it would be a mistake to assume that it can carry the full weight of public health expectations in making non-health focused government departments routinely, systematically, and comprehensively consider the health and well-being impacts of their policies. Emphasis also needs to be placed on allied approaches—both strategic and methodological—that, together with HIA, can increase the level and quality of the consideration of health and wellbeing in policies both nationally and internationally.

In moving the HIA and broader public health in policy agenda forward, Box 7.1 outlines our recommendations for future action.

Box 7.1 Recommendations for how HIA can be more routinely and appropriately used, and how health and wellbeing are considered in national policy making

♦ Departments and ministries of health should give direct and visible support to those government departments that routinely, systematically, and comprehensively consider health and wellbeing impacts.

♦ Recognize the policy constraints and other objectives that government departments have to deliver alongside health, i.e. that health is not the only, or potentially most important, priority and that compromises may be needed to deliver policy interventions that achieve multiple objectives over time.

♦ Explore options and opportunities other than IA for getting health higher on the policy agenda inter-departmentally and inter-ministerially through joint departmental and ministry targets and joint initiatives.

♦ Use inter-departmental and inter-ministerial networks and ambassadors to promote the consideration and analysis of health and wellbeing impacts and HIA.

♦ Provide HIA champions based in departments/ministries of health to help conduct or significantly support the analysis of health and

Box 7.1 (*Continued*)

wellbeing impacts. Alternatively, provide a regular updated online and printed list of public health contacts to help with both the content and process of considering health and wellbeing in policymaking and IAs.

◆ Work with analysts in each government department to develop department-specific approaches and tools to value and quantify health and wellbeing impacts relevant to that department.

◆ Ensure all government departments have strong internal structures that recognize and value health and wellbeing, and an embedded departmental objective on health and wellbeing.

◆ Have high-profile legislation or explicit cabinet/cross-departmental/cross-ministerial support for undertaking HIA that is visibly enforced.

◆ Make policy teams more aware of the wider public health impacts of past and proposed policies through HIA training and other awareness-raising activities, e.g. develop relationships and partnership working with senior civil servants, policy teams, and the department/ministry with responsibility for IA development and monitoring to raise the profile of HIA, to determine what is expected when HIAs are conducted, and to encourage the enforcement of high standards within each government department.

◆ Monitoring by the department/ministry of health and direct and prompt feedback to policy teams in areas where health impacts and the wider determinants of health and health inequalities/equity are not being appropriately considered.

Generic learning points

For public health practitioners and policy-makers

◆ HIA guidance and practice must take into account the practical and political constraints of the policy-making environment.

◆ Unless public health experts contribute to the screening and evidence-gathering stages, it is inevitable that at least some policies with significant health impacts will slip though and not be appropriately analysed

◆ Enable that health and wellbeing are routinely, systematically, and comprehensively considered without creating burdensome bureaucratic requirements is a major challenge.

For educators and researchers

◆ Because of practical and political constraints, there may be a considerable gap between what HIA can add in an ideal policy setting where all policy actors' aims and objectives are aligned and what it can actually add in practice when there are limited resources and multiple, and often conflicting, political and policy agendas.

◆ Even within a compulsory framework it is difficult to overcome the fundamental problem that policy-makers who most need to do HIA are those least likely to undertake it because they see health and wellbeing as not relevant to their policy area.

◆ HIA guidance, no matter how good, is useless if those for whom it is intended are unaware of it or do not use it.

◆ Beyond public health circles, 'health' tends to be narrowly defined. Policymakers can analyse health and wellbeing impacts without describing them as such.

Bibliography

Cabinet Office and Better Regulation Executive (2006) *The tools to deliver better regulation: revising the regulatory impact assessment, a consultation.* London: Better Regulation Executive.

Cole, B.L. and Fielding, J. (2008) *Building health impact assessment (HIA) capacity: a strategy for Congress and Government agencies.* Los Angeles: Partnership for Prevention.

Council for Science and Technology (2006) *Health impacts—a strategy across Government.* London: Council for Science and Technology.

Department of Health (2004) *Policy appraisal and health.* London: Department of Health.

Department of Health (2010a) *Health Impact Assessment of Government Policy: a guide to carrying out a health impact assessment of new policy as part of the impact assessment process.* London: Department of Health.

Department of Health (2010b) *Health Impact Assessment Tools: simple tools for recording the results of health impact assessment.* London: Department of Health.

Department of Health (2010c) *Health Impact Assessment Evidence on Health: a guide to sources of evidence for policymakers carrying out health impact assessment as part of impact assessment of government policy.* London: Department of Health.

Department of Health (2010d) *Quantifying health impacts of government policies: a how-to guide to quantifying the health impacts of government policies.* London: Department of Health.

Department of Health and Institute of Occupational Medicine (2010) *Putting health in the Policy Picture: review of how health impact assessment is carried out by government departments.* Executive Summary. London: Department of Health.

Government of Quebec (2008) *Canadian round table on health impact assessment (HIA). National Collaborating Centre for Healthy Public Policy.* Quebec: National Institute of Public Health.

HM Government (2011a) *Impact Assessment Overview.* London: DBIS.

HM Government (2011b) *Impact Assessment Guidance: when to do an impact assessment.* London: DBIS.

HM Government (2011c) *IA Toolkit: how to do an impact assessment.* London: DBIS.

HM Government (2011d) *Impact Assessment Template.* London: DBIS.

HM Treasury (2011) *The Green Book: appraisal and evaluation in central government.* London: TSO.

Kemm, J. (2006) Health impact assessment and health in all policies, in Stahl, T., Wismar, M., Ollila, E., Lahtinen, E., and Leppo, K. (eds), *Health in all Policies: Prospects and Potentials.* Helsinki: Finnish Ministry of Social Affairs and Health.

Mahoney, M. and Durham, G. (2002) *Health impact assessment: a tool for policy development in Australia.* Faculty of Health and Behavioural Sciences, Melbourne: Deakin University.

NICE (2009) About the HDA. Available at <http://www.nice.org.uk/aboutnice/whoweare/aboutthehda/about_the_hda.jsp>. Accessed 28 March 2012.

Public Health Advisory Committee (2007) *An idea whose time has come: new opportunities for health impact assessment in New Zealand public policy and planning.* Wellington: Public Health Advisory Committee.

The Marmot Review (2010) *Fair Society, Healthy Lives. Strategic Review of Health Inequalities in England post-2010.* London: The Marmot Review.

Varela Put, G., den Broeder, L., Penris, M., and Riscam Abbing, E.W. (2001) *Experience of HIA at national policy level in the Netherlands: a case study.* Policy Learning Curve No. 4. European Centre for Health Policy. Brussels: WHO.

Vohra, S., Amo-Danso, G., and Ball, J. (2011) Further research on how health is considered in England's national policymaking. Unpublished. IOM Centre for Health Impact Assessment, Institute of Occupational Medicine.

Wismar, M., Blau, J., Kelly, E., and Figueras, J. (2007) *The effectiveness of health impact assessment: scope and limitations of supporting decision-making in Europe.* European Observatory on Health Systems and Policies. Trowbridge: The Cromwell Press.

Chapter 8

Health impact assessment in the USA: practice, policy, and legal underpinnings

Catherine L. Ross and Arthi Rao

Introduction

The shift from contagious disease to chronic disease and the realization that health status is influenced by factors beyond traditional healthcare interventions has made clear the need for practical and holistic tools that inform health-related decision-making. The practice of health impact assessment (HIA) has taken root in the USA because it is an effective tool that examines the risk factors, diseases, and equity issues that create poor health outcomes in the USA (Jackson et al. 2011).

Between 1999 and 2007 there were 27 documented HIAs in the USA, indicating a gradual uptake in practice (Dannenberg et al. 2008). In 2011, the Health Impact Project (a collaboration of the Robert Wood Johnson Foundation and the PEW Charitable Trusts) documented 75 completed HIAs in the USA and 40 more in progress. The completed HIAS comprised 11 county (14.7%), 6 federal (8%), 36 local (48%), 6 regional (8%), and 16 state (21.3%) (Health Impact Project 2011). The development of HIA in the USA has been heavily influenced by international theoretical and methodological trends. Integrating health concerns into environmental impact assessment (EIA) and the growth in the field of health promotion, which lists healthy public policy (HPP) and healthy environments among the essential conditions for population health, have been major influences. The types of projects and policies for which HIAs have been conducted vary significantly in both scope and methodology.

Like international models, HIAs in the USA have been conducted as both stand alone and integrated processes with EIAs. Currently, HIA has emerged as a practical platform for catalysing inter-disciplinary collaboration in promoting improved public health. HIA draws on a range of methodologies from the fields of epidemiology, environmental impact analysis, risk analysis, cost-benefit analysis, systematic reviews, and community and transportation planning (Cole and Fielding 2008; Bhatia and Wernham 2006).

HIAs are not legally mandated in the USA and most are conducted on a voluntary basis. However, recent federal strategies such as the *National Prevention Strategy* and *Healthy People 2020* reference HIA as an important tool towards achieving key health outcomes. This strengthens support for the institutionalization of HIA in the future. EIA still remains one of the most established regulatory mechanisms for the incorporation of HIA, but the zone of influence of EIA remains limited, being generally applicable only to federally funded projects. A further critique of current EIA practice is that it assesses health within a very restrictive spectrum mainly defined by biomedical models of health (exposure to toxins, cancer risk). In contrast, HIA resonates with the socio-ecological model of health and includes social determinants of health. In the USA, HIA practice is increasingly encompassing the evaluation of comprehensive planning, transportation improvements, housing and other policies that do not fall into traditional health sectors.

Major actors, institutions, and professions

HIAs in the USA have largely been conducted by public health departments, educational institutions, private organizations, and a number of select institutions. The San Francisco Department of Public Health (SFDPH) has been a leader in the promulgation of HIAs. The University of California Los Angeles School of Public Health, the UCLA Health Impact Assessment Group, Human Impact Partners (HIP) and the Center for Quality Growth and Regional Development (CQGRD) at Georgia Institute of Technology are representative of educational institutions active in the conduct of HIAs. Typically interdisciplinary and organizational partners are formed to conduct HIAs. Examples of these partnerships include the alliance formed to conduct the Atlanta BeltLine, which CQGRD partnered with the Centers for Disease Control and the Robert Woods Johnson Foundation. The Northeast National Petroleum Reserve HIA was conducted through a consortium formed between the US Bureau of Land Management, the Alaska Intertribal Council and the Columbia University Institute on Medicine as a Profession. The following list includes both public and private entities active in HIA funding and practice:

- Annie E. Casey Foundation
- Blue Cross/Blue Shield of Minnesota Foundation
- California Endowment
- Centers for Disease Control and Prevention
- Ford Foundation

- Health Impact Project (Robert Wood Johnson and Pew Charitable Trusts)
- Hewlett Foundation
- Kresge Foundation
- Liberty Hill
- National Institute of Environmental Health Sciences
- Northwest Health Foundation
- Public Welfare Foundation
- Robert Wood Johnson Foundation
- WK Kellogg Foundation.

Funding is available through grants from federal state and private/non-profit agencies. Federal programmes similar to Communities Putting Prevention to Work and grants made by the Department of Housing and Urban Development/ Department of Transportation/Environmental Protection Agency (HUD/ DOT/EPA) Sustainable Communities effort specifically identify HIA as an approved activity.

Examples of current HIA practice

The two HIAs described in the following sections are examples of HIA diversity in the USA, with one focusing on policy and the other on a project.

The Unhealthy Consequences: Energy Costs and Child Health HIA

The Unhealthy Consequences: Energy Costs and Child Health HIA addressed the health risks for low-income children associated with unaffordable energy costs and the Low Income Home Energy Assistance Program (LIHEAP). This federally funded programme is designed to help low-income families heat their homes. The Department of Pediatrics at Boston Medical Center and Boston University School of Medicine convened an inter-disciplinary working group to develop a child health impact assessment (CHIA) strategy in 2004. They conceptualized the CHIA as analogous to an EIA. The goal of the CHIA was to evaluate the impacts of regulations and laws on children's health and wellbeing, with a particular focus on policy areas outside the traditional realm of public health.

The CHIA analysis used previously collected data and best available scientific evidence. The type of data collected included academic and other research, government databases, advocacy websites, and interviews with key stakeholders. The CHIA working group collected information on LIHEAP, home energy costs, and their effects on a child's basic needs, including education, housing, food, access to health care, safety and stability, and the physical environment.

The HIA included the valuation of trade-offs families make between paying energy bills and other needs, including the purchase of food or clothing, referred to as 'heat or eat', and the health risks that result when families rely on unhealthy or unsafe heating sources when they cannot pay heating bills or move to substandard housing. The HIA also assessed other health risks—such as burns and carbon monoxide poisoning—that can result when families use unsafe heating sources. Finally, they identified the unhealthy living conditions faced by families who were no longer able to afford adequate housing because of high energy costs, e.g. exposure to pests, water leaks and mould, peeling lead paint, and the resulting health hazards. The study focused on the 400,000 children in Massachusetts.

The group employed a measure developed within the US Department of Health and Human Services, which administers the LIHEAP. It is a reliable, easy-to-use tool that evaluates the impact of energy costs on a family. The Home Energy Insecurity Scale makes it possible to capture all aspects of low income affordability: thriving, capable, stable, vulnerable, and in crisis. The CHIA documents that unaffordable energy costs adversely affect the health of low-income children and have potential consequences on health that are preventable.

HIA of the BeltLine: Atlanta's emerald necklace

The BeltLine is a transformative project shaping the way Atlanta will mature, by creating parks, trails, transit, and a new development along a 22-mile loop of historic rail segments that encircle the city's urban core (Figure 8.1). This ambitious redevelopment is transforming Atlanta into a city connected by transit, trails, and green space, with significant health benefits. The project costs are estimated to be approximately $3 billion. The revival of this historically industrial landscape can potentially serve as an exemplary national model for the integration of health in redevelopment. How do we understand the health impacts of a new development? To answer this question for the Atlanta BeltLine project, CQGRD conducted an HIA (Ross C.L., 2007). The BeltLine HIA is one of the first in the USA that elevated the discussion of health impacts to a regional level when the BeltLine was ranked highly as a project with regional significance. The HIA was completed in 2007. It was a prospective study and health impacts as assessed have influenced implementation decisions around the BeltLine. Using content analysis of over 3 years of newspaper articles, a public survey, literature review, and professional expertise, the research team

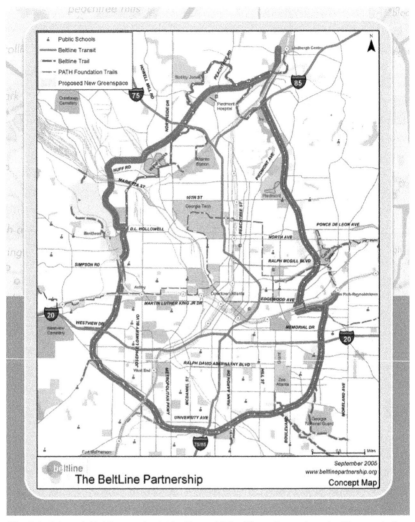

Fig. 8.1 Atlanta's Beltline project, the Emerald Necklace. Reproduced with permission of Atlanta BeltLine. Copyright © 2012 Atlanta BeltLine, All Rights Reserved.

identified several critical issues that have the potential to impact the health of the study area population. These include access to amenities, goods, and services, opportunities for physical activity, social capital, safety, and environmental issues such as air quality, water management, noise, and brownfields.

The Atlanta Beltline HIA research team consisted of multi-disciplinary researchers (composed largely of staff of the CDC, Georgia Institute of Technology Faculty, and researchers) with expertise in public health and planning. An advisory committee was recruited to provide overall project direction, component-specific guidance, and analytical expertise. A priority of the BeltLine HIA was the assessment of potential health impacts on the most vulnerable members of the study area population. The potentially vulnerable populations were individuals with low economic status, children, older adults, renters, and the carless. A variety of methodologies and data sources were used including, but not limited to, census data, travel data, latent demand analysis, walkability audits, quality growth audits, interviews, surveys and public outreach methods, and air and noise analysis.

The research team measured changes in equitable access to parks and trails, transportation, healthy housing, and healthy food. For access to parks, Geographic Information System (GIS) analysis examined existing and proposed parkland. Researchers calculated the percentage of residents who had park access now and in 2030, and their composition by age, race, income, poverty or carless status, and planning subarea. Thirteen per cent of the residents in the BeltLine study area did not have access to a park prior to the BeltLine project. The analysis showed that park access would increase for study area residents and for the city of Atlanta. Investigators recommended that the BeltLine should increase physical activity by prioritizing construction of greenspace and pedestrian access to transit, incorporating universal design principles to enable and encourage the elderly, people with disabilities, and children to use the facilities, and providing lighting and emergency infrastructure to increase the perceived safety of the facilities. A testament to the effectiveness of the HIA is that it is being adopted as a primary assessment tool by Beltline Inc. The Beltline HIA is also referenced as a primary reason for the investment of $6 million thus far in additional funding from the public and private sector, and the rating of the project as the highest priority for the Atlanta metro region.

Legal foundation of HIA

Beginning in the 1950s, social activism and ecological thought ('everything is connected to everything else') heavily influenced environmental thought. Concerns over environmental toxins and impacts on humans as well as animals prompted environmental action in the 1960s. Economic and industrial development was also creating large-scale pollution of rivers, streams, and coastlines. In response, the Federal government passed NEPA in 1969. In the interest of environmental justice, NEPA mandated public participation in the land development process (Kuzmiak 1991) to minimize environmental impacts and to assure more equitable distribution of positive outcomes between populations.

During the 1970s, there were several policy changes: the Environmental Protection Agency (EPA) was created and key federal legislation such as the Clean Air Act (regulates hazardous air pollutant emissions from stationary and mobile sources by establishing National Ambient Air Quality Standards), the Clean Water Act (establishes similar standards for water quality by regulating contamination from wastewater and industrial pollutants), and the Occupational Safety and Health Act were passed.

The US legal framework and HIA

NEPA marks the legal origin of the EIA as an 'operational tool to guide planning and decision-making having an impact on the quality of environment and the health and safety of the people' and a legal tool to enforce environmental sensitivity in policy decisions (Caldwell 1988: 78). NEPA and related state laws mandate the identification and analysis of health effects when an EIA is conducted. EIA, however, has traditionally included only a perfunctory analysis of health impacts (Corburn 2004; Steinemann 2000, Vanclay and Bronstein,1995). Some argue that health analysis should be integrated into EIA because NEPA and related state laws provide a mechanism for achieving the same goals as HIA. Others suggest that the independence of HIA is critical to its effectiveness, which might be diminished through integration (Cole et al, 2004; Cole et al, 2005). The appropriate assessment of health effects in EIA under NEPA is required by law; HIA can be integrated into NEPA in compliance with existing legal requirements. On the other hand, states such as Massachusetts have mandated the HIA requirement for all transportation-related projects as part of their Transportation Reform Act, lending credence to it as a standalone process.

Twenty states and US territories have now enacted regional versions of NEPA laws. Each year more than 500 environmental impact statements are completed at the federal level, as are thousands of similar assessments under state-level environmental assessment laws. Many decisions guided by these assessments present an excellent opportunity to protect and improve public health (Jackson et al. 2011).

Early attempts involved the incorporation of HIA into the procedural requirements of EIA. HIAs modelled on EIAs are referred to as 'narrow' or 'tight' models focused on projects and methodologies influenced by biomedical models of health. 'Broad' models are more characteristic of HIAs that examine policies rather than projects (Cole and Fielding 2007). Nevertheless, the major task is to establish empirically based pathways between social, economic, and environmental links to human health.

Barriers to the institutionalization of HIA

A major challenge for HIA is that it is not legally mandated. EIA still remains one of the most established regulatory mechanisms (as exemplified by the practice of HIA in Alaska). Recent initiatives such as the federal Sustainable Communities Initiative recognize the creation of healthy communities as a vital goal. The Federal Interagency Working Group established in 1994 requires that federal programmes consider policies for improving environmental quality and public health for vulnerable populations among other environmental justice considerations (CEQ 1997). This provides a wider, more upstream platform for the incorporation of mandatory HIA language within existing legal frameworks. However, knowledge of existing laws and statutes that could support the incorporation of HIA remains limited. Further research is required to understand the wide array of federal, tribal, state, and local laws that favour or include health considerations. Additional needs and barriers to the institutionalization of HIA include greater capacity building, the need for greater analytic and financial resources, data collection, more evidence-based HIAs, cross-disciplinary training, and greater integration of HIA into NEPA, (Dannenberg et al. 2006; Cole and Fielding 2008; Rajotte et al. 2011).

Generic learning points

For public health practitioners and policy-makers

- The development of multi-disciplinary and multi-sectorial teams is critical to the conduct of high-quality evidence-based HIAs that influence decision outcomes. Many of the factors affecting health originate outside the realm of public health and HIA offers a promising opportunity to engage sectors outside of public health.

- Expanding the role of government agencies and decision-makers in efforts to improve public health requires practical tools that integrate HIA into decision-making and in the development of regulations and plans.

- Government agencies, including health departments, should seek funding from traditional sources, including permit fees, development fees, and corporative agreements on cost sharing and partnerships with the private sector, to overcome financial constraints. The creation of legislation to mandate and fund the conduct of HIAs (only the state of Massachusetts has done this to date) is one avenue being developed. Engagement with multi-disciplinary partners outside the health sector, including planning departments, public works departments, departments of natural resources, and development authorities, provides additional funding opportunities.

- ◆ Working partnerships between the local community, voluntary sector, key service providers, authorities, and decision-makers is critical to increasing the awareness of HIA.
- ◆ Recent efforts in the USA have demonstrated that projects, policies, or programmes can be modified to improve health outcomes without a major change in the existing environment.
- ◆ HIA practice can be expanded by conducting HIAs in new and evolving areas.
- ◆ The effectiveness and benefits of the HIA may not be immediately obvious since projects can cover a span of many years. In these instances, HIA can be effective in improving the process or expanding long-term collaboration while awaiting achievement of its primary purpose.

For educators and researchers

- ◆ The development of a more explicit focus and research agenda on 'population health' as a function of the non-medical determinants of health can be a primary tool to improve the receptivity of HIA. This approach could figure prominently in research priorities as a strategy to develop a more conducive environment for HIA.
- ◆ A primary need is to improve the receptivity of HIA and one strategy is the development of a more explicit focus and research agenda on 'population health' as a function of the non-medical determinants of health. This approach could figure prominently in research priorities as a strategy to develop a more conducive environment for HIA.
- ◆ Training and capacity building remain outstanding challenges to the promulgation of HIAs. Educational institutions and professional societies must expand activity and productivity through increased offerings of training modules that are appropriate for a broad spectrum from community organizations to professionals. Effective HIA practice requires wide knowledge-based inter-disciplinary curriculum development.
- ◆ Systematic HIA evaluation to determine overall effectiveness is often ignored or based on informal/biased self-reports from practitioners. Creating rigorous methods for evaluation is an important research need. Standards must be addressed to gauge the benefit and effectiveness of HIA and promote it as a comprehensive multi-disciplinary tool for integrating health outcomes into everyday decision-making.

References

Bhatia, R. and Wernham, A. (2008) Integrating human health into environmental impact assessment: an unrealized opportunity for environmental health and justice. *Environmental Health Perspectives* 116 (8): 1159–1175.

Caldwell, L.K. (1988) Environmental impact analysis (EIA): origins, evolution, and future directions. *Review of Policy Research* 8 (1): 75–83.

Child Health Impact Working Group (2007) *Unhealthy Consequences: Energy Costs and Child Health.* Available at <http://www.healthimpactproject.org/resources/document/massachusetts-low-income-energy-assistance-program.pdf>.

Cole, B.L. and Fielding, J.E. (2007) Health impact assessment: a tool to help policy makers understand health beyond health care. *Annual Review of Public Health* 28: 393–412.

Cole, B.L. and Fielding, J.E. (2008) Building health impact assessment (HIA) capacity: a strategy for congress and government agencies: a prevention policy paper commissioned by partnership for prevention. Washington DC: Partnership for Prevention. Available at http://www.prevent.org/data/files/initiatives/buildignhealthimpactassessmenthiacapacity.pdf.

Cole, B.L, Wilhelm M., et al. (2004) Prospects for health impact assessment in the United States: new and improved environmental impact assessment or something different? *Journal of Health Politics, Policy, and Law* 29 (6): 1153–1186.

Cole, B.L., Shimkhada, R., Fielding, J., Kominski, G., and Morgenstern, H. (2005) Methodologies for realizing the potential of health impact assessment. *American Journal of Preventive Medicine* 28(4): 382–389.

Corburn, J. (2004) Confronting the challenges in reconnecting urban planning and public health. *American Journal of Public Health* 94 (4): 541–549.

(1997) Environmental Justice: Guidance under theNational Environmental Quality Act. Washington, DC: Council on Environmental Quality. Available at <http://www.epa.gov/environmentaljustice/resources/policy/ej_guidance_nepa_ceq1297.pdf>.

Dannenberg, A.L., Bhatia, R., Cole, B.L., Dora, C., Fielding, J.E., Kraft, K., et al. (2006) Growing the field of health impact assessment in the United States: an agenda for research and practice. *American Journal of Public Health* 96 (2): 262–270.

Dannenberg, A.L., Bhatia, R., Cole, B.L., Heaton, S.K., Feldman, J.D., and Rutt, C.D. (2008) Use of health impact assessment in the US: 27 case studies, 1999–2007. *American Journal of Preventive Medicine* 34 (3): 241–256.

Health Impact Project (2011) *HIA in the United States.* Available at <http://www.health-impactproject.org/hia/us>.

Jackson, R., Bear, D., Bhatia, R., Cantor, S.B., Cave, B., Diez Roux, A.V., Dora, C., Fielding, J.E., Zivin, J.S.G., Levy, J.I., Quint, J.I., Raja, S., Schulz, A.J., and Wernham, A.A. (2011) *Improving Health in the United States: The Role of Health Impact Assessment.* Washington, DC: Committee on Health Impact Assessment. Board on Environmental Studies and Toxicology, Division on Earth and Life Studies, National Research Council of the National Academies. Available at <http://www.nap.edu/catalog.php?record_id=13229>. Accessed 5 July 2012.

Kuzmiak, D. (1991) The American environmental movement. *Geographical Journal* 157 (3): 265–278.

National Research Council (2011) *Improving Health in the United States: The Role of Health Impact Assessment*. Washington, DC: The National Academies Press.

Rajotte, B., Ross, C., Ekechi, C., and Cadet, V. (2011) Health in all policies: addressing the legal and policy foundations of health impact assessment. *Journal of Law, Medicine & Ethics* 39: 27–29.

Ross, C.L. (2007) *Atlanta BeltLine Health Impact Assessment*. Center for Quality Growth and Regional Development, Georgia Institute of Technology, Atlanta, GA.

Steinemann, A. (2000) Rethinking human health impact assessment. *Environmental Impact Assessment Review* 20: 627–645.

Vanclay, F. and Bronstein, D.(1995) *Environmental and Social Impact Assessment*. Brisbane: Wiley and Sons.

Chapter 9

'Learning by doing'—building workforce capacity to undertake health impact assessment: an Australian case study

Elizabeth Harris, Ben Harris-Roxas, Patrick Harris, and Lynn Kemp

Introduction

There has been a longstanding interest in Australia in developing health impact assessment (HIA) as an effective way of assessing the impact of policies, programmes, and projects on health. Between 2000 and 2004 the Australian federal government funded two HIA-related programmes through its Public Health Education and Research Program. The first was undertaken by Mary Mahoney and Gillian Durham and made a case for the use of HIA in policy development in Australia (Mahoney and Durham 2002). Rosemary Aldrich et al. developed a framework for undertaking equity focused health impact assessment (EFHIA) that involved a literature review (Harris-Roxas et al. 2004) and piloted the framework with five case studies (Simpson et al. 2005).

Background

Buoyed by growing interest in undertaking HIA in the UK and Europe, and the importance given to routinely considering equity within the HIA process, the New South Wales Health and Equity Statement *In All Fairness* (NSW Health 2004) recommended HIA as a key organizational development strategy to increase the NSW health system's capacity to address health inequities. It was recognized that health workforce and organizational capacity to conduct HIAs required development in order to implement the *In All Fairness* recommendations. To build these capacities, the NSW Department of Health funded what was eventually to be a three-phase programme. In this chapter the focus will be on one aspect of the capacity building programme—its workforce development strategies, specifically 'learning by doing' (LbD).

Case study: the NSW HIA Programme

The broad purpose of phases 1 and 2 of the NSW HIA Programme (the Programme) was to explore the feasibility and mechanisms for the development of HIA processes in NSW, and to increase awareness in the NSW health system of the purpose and potential uses for HIA. The Centre for Health Equity Training, Research and Evaluation (CHETRE) at the University of New South Wales (UNSW) was contracted to undertake the Programme. In phase 1 (2002–2003) discussions and a number of information sessions on HIA were held with key stakeholders within the health system. It became apparent that unless there was a body of experience in undertaking HIA in NSW many of the reservations expressed could not be addressed, such as the lack of a robust evidence base, scepticism that HIA would be effective in influencing policy, project and programmes, and unwillingness by area health services and other parts of the health system to redirect limited resources to HIA.

Phases 2 and 3 focused on building capacity through providing the health workforce with practical experiences in undertaking HIA, through implementation of collaborative project-based learning opportunities. Colloquially known as 'learning by doing', this is an effective process for the creation of the four levels of knowledge needed to undertake complex, collaborative, technical, and value-based activities such as HIA (Tilchin 2011):

- ◆ know-what (cognitive knowledge)
- ◆ know-how (procedural knowledge)
- ◆ know-why (theoretical knowledge)
- ◆ care-why (situational/social knowledge).

Project-based learning (in this context LbD) has two aims: firstly the 'creation and acquisition of knowledge within a project' and secondly the subsequent codification and transfer of such knowledge to other parts of the organization (Scarbrough et al. 2004; Poell et al. 2009; Bakker and Cambre et al. 2011). It is well recognized that achievement of the second aim can be problematic. Once the project is completed, participants 'can struggle to translate the learning into practice in their localized settings' (Poell et al. 2009).

The LbD strategy was thus embedded within a range of capacity building interventions informed by the NSW Health Capacity Building Framework. This framework proposes five key action areas where change needs to occur: organizational development, workforce development, resource allocation, partnerships, and leadership. Over time these were cross-referenced with action that needed to be taken at local, meso (often regional), and macro level (usually state or national levels—see Table 9.1). Developing organizational capacity was therefore seen as a complex, multilevel task. Other workforce development strategies included development of a three-day elective course as part of the Master of Public Health at UNSW, short courses in HIA, conference and workshops presentations, organizing an international conference and colloquium, peer-reviewed publications, a regular electronic newsletter, and the HIA Connect website.

LbD strategy

Four rounds of LbD were undertaken between 2004 and 2007. A total of 19 HIAs were supported by the LbD process (an average of five per year).

Table 9.1 An example of the use of the NSW Capacity Building Framework to improve workforce capacity

Type of intervention	Local	Meso	Macro
Organizational development	Commitment to LbD	Requirement for all major policies to undergo HIA or EFHIA	Strategic commitment to and ongoing mechanisms for conducting HIA
Workforce development	Staff participation in LbD strategy	Training programmes and professional placements	Consistent funding to support LbD strategy
Resource development	Posting on website, dissemination of LbD projects	Providing access to internet to allow access to resources	HIA manual and resources for HIA such as evidence reviews
Partnerships	Inter-organizational LbD projects	Developing ongoing inter-organizational regional collaborations	Align HIA with other planning processes and IAs
Leadership	Inter-organizational LbD projects	Annual showcase and awards	Identify and support inter-organizational 'champions'

The majority of HIAs were undertaken as intermediate, requiring some additional data collection (Harris et al. 2007) and, consistent with the brief to build health system capacity, the majority of HIAs (10) were related to health services and programmes, four HIAs were concerned with land use planning and development in the built environment, and five with local and regional strategic and population planning.

The LbD strategy consisted of an eight-stage process. The strengths and challenges in undertaking the LbD strategy are discussed below.

Proposal identification

Initially the HIA team would only accept proposals that were well-developed, well-documented, and where there was still an opportunity to influence decisions. However, it soon became apparent that in many policies, plans, and programmes there was no clear point at which the proposal was detailed yet still able to be influenced. For example, once a policy was drafted and had been reviewed by relevant stakeholders it was often not feasible, and unpopular, to try and change it. On the other hand, if the proposal was underdeveloped it was difficult to screen and particularly to scope it in a way that made it possible to undertake a timely and focused assessment. We have found some resistance within the health system in undertaking HIA as practitioners believe positive and negative health impacts have already been identified in their planning process and adequately addressed. LbD is most successful where the project is of high importance, is a significant and urgent problem, and is the team's responsibility to solve (Yeo and Nation, 2010; Kinsey 2011). There was more support for undertaking EFHIAs, particularly closer to the implementation phase, as there was an acceptance that equity may have been poorly addressed in prior planning.

An expression of interest (EOI) process was undertaken because of the limited capacity of CHETRE to support more than four to six HIAs at any one time. This involved identifying the proposal, who would be involved in the project team, and why it was considered important. These EOIs were then assessed by an independent panel (including a representative of CHETRE) against these criteria with follow-up phone contact or interviews if clarification was needed. This process was valuable in helping to assess if the HIA was feasible and likely to be completed. There was usually a match between the number of HIAs we could support and those that were accepted through the EOI process.

In addition to the participants that were in the HIA team we also developed a process for 'participant observers'. These observers were generally from an organization other than those in the HIA team, and had a strong interest in learning about HIA but did not have a developed proposal to work on. Observers were partnered with specific LbD HIA teams and were expected to attend all training sessions, where feasible attend screening and scoping meetings, and undertake some aspect of data collection. Generally each LbD HIA team had one participant observer.

Written support from senior staff

In order to put forward an EOI each team had to provide a letter of support from the Chief Executive Officer of the local area health service (AHS) that committed the organization to allowing staff to attend training and undertake the HIA. This was initially thought to ensure adequate support for the HIA, be an indication of the organization's commitment to the project and valuing of the project as 'real work', and a marker of potential to embed the learning into organizational systems, structures, procedures, and strategy (Scarbrough et al. 2004; Swan et al. 2010). This was in part true but unfortunately most participants had to incorporate the HIA into their existing workload. As CHETRE were all inexperienced we underestimated the time that would be needed to undertake what were generally intermediate HIAs. We also did not foresee the wide-reaching changes to the structures in AHSs and changes in senior management that would impact on the roles of participants and the opportunities to embed HIA practice in AHSs. This involved merging 16 AHSs into eight, merging senior roles so there was only one senior position in each AHS (where there previously been two), rationalizing the location of service into larger groupings, and coping with cultural and organizational issues that existed between AHS and the HIA program.

Because participants were required to undertake training to participate in the programme initially it was decided that three to five days of formal training were required. Each HIA team nominated two to four people to attend training (initially these people were largely from health services but over time included representatives from other sectors and community groups). The content and method of delivery developed over time. Today LbD training is ideally provided in three sessions (two days, two days, one day) generally over four to six months:

◆ Days 1–2: Overview of HIA, the steps of HIA, and screening and scoping

◆ Days 3–4: Identification and assessment of impacts, negotiation, and decision-making

◆ Day 5: Evaluation and presentation on progress to date

Participants found the opportunity to work on their projects and discuss common problems very useful. One strength of LbD was the involvement of rural areas in training. Funding was provided for two people from each rural site to attend all sessions of the LbD training by paying for their travel and accommodation.

Site visits

To ensure the HIA teams were adequately supported, each project was allocated a CHETRE programme team member as a 'coach' to aid their learning. Site visits were organized where the CHETRE coach met with HIA team, the steering committee, or other stakeholders to clarify their roles, the process, and the outcomes of their involvement. Where possible the site visits were undertaken prior to training and at two other critical periods of the HIA. These site visits were invaluable for the HIA project team and CHETRE programme team as it made the nature of the proposal and local context clear and also indicated to participants that CHETRE understood the context and resource constraints under which they were working.

Help desk support

The evaluation of the project highlighted the importance of help desk support as one of the most valuable aspects of the project. Each team was able to and encouraged to contact the CHETRE programme team if they needed support. Where possible the CHETHRE 'coach' taking the lead on visits to the site was also the primary contact for help desk support. Help desk support covered a wide variety of issues, including technical assistance on specific steps, advice on engaging members of the steering committee, sources of evidence of potential impacts, referral to other similar HIAs, writing up, and preparation of presentations and publications. The help desk support was provided through phone calls and emails.

Resources

The development of the HIA manual, screening tools, resources on the HIA Connect website, newsletters, and listserves was seen by participants as a key aspect in supporting the HIA process. The HIA team did not fully appreciate the importance of the website and list serves as a way of connecting projects in and outside the LbD process.

Preparation of peer-reviewed publications and conference presentations

One component of workforce development is building capacity to contribute to knowledge in the field. This was done by encouraging and assisting participants to prepare papers for peer-reviewed publications and make presentations at conferences. The 2007 inaugural Asia Pacific HIA Conference was part of the NSW HIA Program and it has led to three subsequent Asia Pacific conferences in Chiang Mai, Dunedin, and Seoul, providing opportunities for conference presentations at national and international conferences.

Finalization of HIA report and posting on website

All teams were required to complete a full HIA report that would be uploaded to the HIA Connect website. This was often a long and time-consuming process as once the pressure to complete the HIA was past, participants' focus returned to their core responsibility. Projects are usually temporary, finite, and unique in nature, and it is likely that following completion of the project participants move on (or back) to other (or regular) work (Poell et al. 2009; Swan et al. 2010). Project completion may thus also lead to 'learning closure' (Scarbrough et al. 2004). Posting reports on the website was a strategy for institutionalizing the learning, or knowledge codification, whereby the knowledge can be accessed and used by others (Swan et al. 2010).

Box 9.1 Reflections by participants on LbD

The strength of the LbD approach is based on three case studies from the independent evaluation of phase 3 HIIA project.

The HIA training and LbD methodology was regarded as a key strength of the project by almost every participant. Participants commented that the training was:

+ logical, proceeded through successive steps, linked theory to practice

+ effective in linking staff from other departments within health and to partners outside of health to learn together, share ideas, and develop skills.

The LbD methodology was regarded as a critical factor in integrating HIA within AHSs.

Evaluation

In the final independent evaluation of the capacity building programme in 2008, LbD was identified as a major success (Quigley and Watts Ltd 2008). Box 9.1 summarizes the evaluation of the LbD strategy from two case studies. CHETRE also received the IAIA Institutional Award in 2010 in recognition of its HIA capacity building work.

Case study 1: Rural area health service

One participant regarded the training provided by CHETRE as a strength. This person thought it was logical, proceeded through successive steps, and provided a grounding in how to undertake an HIA in practice. The training also provided an opportunity for staff from other departments within the AHS and external partners to learn together, share knowledge, and develop skills. The LbD approach, although sometimes challenging, was regarded by some participants as the most useful way to learn HIA.

Case study 2: Urban redevelopment LbD team

The CHETRE project's ground-up capacity building approach was seen as being responsible for the achievements that have been made. The LbD approach and working within the developmental sites was seen as an important contributor to these achievements.

Sustainability

There have been some signs that capacity has been sustained beyond of the funding of the NSW HIA Programme. Since the finalization of the Programme we have supported a further 11 HIAs with funding from health services in NSW, South Australia, and Queensland, government departments in NSW and other Australian states, and a number of non-government organizations. There have also been one advocacy and two community-led HIAs. A third of all HIAs have been EFHIAs. Continued implementation of HIA projects within the core work setting has been particularly strong in health services where there is a critical mass of people who have participated in the LbD programme (Poell et al. 2009), that is, where there is sufficient 'experience accumulation' (Swan et al. 2010) and, in the case of intersectoral HIA projects, where there is ongoing collaboration (Swan et al. 2010; Bakker et al. 2011).

Competency in HIA has been included in the NSW Public Health Officer Training Programme and there continues to be strong support for training through an HIA unit within the UNSW Master of Public Health programme and an annual professional development course. We are training and supporting HIA in four other states, through LbD in Far North Queensland and training programmes in Tasmania, Northern Territory, and Western Australia. CHETRE has also conducted training programmes in Korea, Thailand, and most recently for WHO for the Americas (participants from over 20 countries in the Americas). Later in 2012 a training course will be held in Mexico sponsored by the American Chapter of the International Union of Health Promotion and Education.

Generic learning points

LbD has proven to be an effective, popular, and sustainable way of improving health system capacity to undertake HIA.

Although this work has helped to raise awareness and seen the adoption of HIA by some champions of innovation, much still needs to be done in reorienting the health system to include HIA in mainstream population health practice.

For public health practitioners and policy-makers

◆ Workforce development should be seen as only one component of efforts to build capacity to undertake HIA. Organizational support and investment in resources are also needed. Training in undertaking HIA will have limited traction if staff are expected to build HIA into their current responsibilities or if there is no mechanism for the findings of the HIA to be considered by decision makers.

◆ It is often difficult to judge when is the best time to undertake an HIA as there was no clear point at which the proposal was detailed enough to undertake an HIA and yet still be able to be influenced.

◆ Building organizational capacity to undertake HIA requires attention to the level of organizational support and infrastructure for the HIA process.

◆ As well as focus on a skilled workforce, adequate resources, especially time, are required. The best way to learn about HIA is by doing one.

For educators and researchers

◆ Competence in undertaking HIA requires active learning by doing an HIA in a real-world setting wherever possible.

◆ LbD is one way of doing this that involves training, site visits, help desk support, report preparation, and presentation of findings.

Acknowledgements

As well as the authors of this paper, the LbD initiative was the product of the work and collaboration of several people, including Sarah Simpson, former project manager for the NSW HIA Capacity Building Program, CHETRE, Hannah Baird, Mary Mahoney, Jenny Hughes, and Caron Bowen. We would also like to acknowledge all those who participated in the LbD programme over the years.

References

Bakker, R.M., Cambre, B., Korlaar, L., and Raab, J. (2011) Managing the project learning paradox: a set-theoretic approach toward project knowledge transfer. *International Journal of Project Management* 29: 494–503.

Harris, P., Harris-Roxas, B., Harris, E., and Kemp, L. (2007) Health impact assessment: a practical guide,Centre for Health Equity Training, part of the UNSW Research Centre for Primary Health Care and Equity. Sydney: UNSW.

Harris-Roxas, B.F., Simpson, S., and Harris, E. (2004) *Equity Focussed Health Impact Assessment: A Literature Review.* Sydney: Centre for Health Equity Training, Research and Evaluation, University of New South Wales.

Kinsey, S.B. (2011) Action learning—an experiential tool for solving organizational issues. *Journal of Extension* 49 (4): 4TOT2.

Mahoney, M. and Durham, G. (2002) *Health Impact Assessment: a tool for policy development in Australia, Report for Commonwealth Department for Health and Ageing.* Melbourne: Deakin University.

NSW Health (2004) *NSW Health and Equity Statement: In All Fairness.* Sydney: NSW Department of Health.

Poell, R.F., Yorks, L., and Marsick, V.J. (2009) Organizing project-based learning in work contexts: a cross-cultural analysis of data from two projects. *Adult Education Quarterly* 60 (1): 77–93.

Quigley and Watts Ltd (2008) *Evaluation of Phase Three of the New South Wales Health Impact Assessment Project: Final Report.* Sydney: Quigley and Watts for the Centre for Health Equity Training Research and Evaluation, Research Centre for Primary Health Care and Equity, UNSW.

Scarbrough, H., Bresnen, M., Edelman, L.F., Laurent, S., Newell, S., and Swan, J. (2004) The processes of project-based learning: an exploratory study. *Management Learning* 35 (4): 491–506.

Simpson, S., Mahoney, M., Harris, E., Aldrich, R., and Stewart-Williams, J. (2005) Equity-focused health impact assessment: A tool to assist policy makers in addressing health inequalities. *Environmental Impact Assessment Review* 25 (7–8): 772–782.

Swan, J., Scarbrough, H., and Newell, S. (2010) Why don't (or do) organizations learn from projects? *Management Learning* 41 (3): 325–344.

Tilchin, O. (2011) Promotion of knowledge building during learning by doing. *Intenational Journal of Learning* 17 (1): 473–493.

Yeo, R.K., and Nation, U.E. (2010) Optimizing the action in action learning: urgent problems, diversified group membership, and commitment to action. *Advances in Developing Human Resources* 12 (2): 181–204.

Chapter 10

Health impact assessment in local government: a New Zealand case study

Louise Signal, Matthew Soeberg, and Robert Quigley

Introduction

Since 2005 there has been a substantial increase in the number of health impact assessments (HIAs) undertaken in New Zealand, largely at the local level. This chapter presents the New Zealand case and critically reflects on the strengths and weaknesses of the New Zealand approach. The chapter is based on a review of New Zealand literature, documentary analysis of completed HIA reports and evaluations, and the knowledge of the authors.

Context

In late 2011, 47 HIAs were completed or in progress in New Zealand. Multiple factors contributed to this number, including the focus on determinants of health and health inequalities, and New Zealand's legal, procedural, and political context.

Determinants of health and health inequalities

New Zealand's constitutional arrangements were important in the development of HIA, specifically the need to address ethnic and socio-economic health inequalities. The Treaty of Waitangi is the foundation document for New Zealand and articulates the rights and responsibilities of Māori (the indigenous population comprising about 15% of the total New Zealand population) and the New Zealand government. The Treaty has special relevance to Māori health as breaches of the Treaty have impacted on the economic, social, and physical conditions in which Māori live. Furthermore, the Treaty ensures that Māori have the same right to health as non-Māori. Finally, the Treaty has relevance to the planning and delivery of healthcare services in New Zealand requiring them to protect and promote Māori health and wellbeing.

The election of a centre-left government in 1999 saw the introduction of substantial health reforms, including the establishment of the district health board (DHB) system. DHBs are largely responsible for the funding and provision of healthcare and public health services in their regions. They are required to improve the health of their populations and to reduce health inequalities. Alongside this were the *New Zealand Health Strategy* (Minister of Health 2000) and a strategy for reducing health inequalities (Ministry of Health 2002), both of which provided an important entry point for HIA. Furthermore, the New Zealand evidence base on the importance of addressing the determinants of health was building through the work of the National Health Committee, an independent advisory committee to the Minister of Health (National Health Committee 1998).

Legal, procedural, and political factors

Changes in local government legislation have been critical in progressing HIA. Local government has an important role in the provision of public health services in New Zealand, although much public health activity is led by DHB public health units. Core activities of local government include water and sanitation, resource management, and refuse collection. In addition, local government leads or supports other public health activities such as providing or facilitating access to community services. The local government role in broader public health activities was formalized by the Local Government Act 2002, which required local councils to develop policies to promote social, economic, environmental, and cultural wellbeing. The inclusion of these four wellbeings extended the formal scope of local government work and provided public health with an additional entry point. Furthermore, new legal frameworks in areas such as building and transport had explicit requirements for protecting and promoting public health and implications for local government. Protecting air and water quality, and regional transport planning are the responsibility of regional councils, an area of some HIA activity.

The procedural framework for HIA was also core to its rapid development. A turning point was the 2004 publication of policy-level HIA guidelines by the Public Health Advisory Committee (PHAC), a subcommittee of the National Health Committee (Public Health Advisory Committee 2004). The Ministry of Health released additional HIA guidelines in 2007 that provided greater focus on whānau ora (health and wellbeing for Māori, their families and communities) (Ministry of Health 2007). HIAs undertaken within New Zealand's environmental framework are discussed elsewhere (Morgan 2008).

The need to expand HIA practice across New Zealand also gained political traction. Based on evaluations of HIAs undertaken around 2005, for example

Quigley and Burt (2006), the executive arm of the New Zealand government agreed in 2006 to establish a national HIA Support Unit within the Ministry of Health.

New Zealand case study

Table 10.1 shows the HIAs completed or in progress in New Zealand since 2005, which span a range of health determinants and proposal types. Based on Mahoney et al.'s (2004) classification, the majority have been of intermediate size. All were voluntary as there is no legislative requirement to undertake them. Most were done on a limited budget, often with tight timeframes, by relatively inexperienced practitioners supported by experienced consultants. All but two have been prospective.

The Draft Greater Christchurch Urban Development Strategy (UDS) HIA, one of the best evaluated New Zealand HIAs, is explained in more detail below. Recently, Christchurch has been severely affected by a series of earthquakes that have meant a complete re-examination of urban development in the region.

Draft Greater Christchurch Urban Development Strategy HIA

The Draft Greater Christchurch UDS (Urban Development Forum 2004) was a high-level planning document to guide urban growth in the Greater Christchurch region over the following 40 years. It was produced by several local government authorities and the New Zealand Transport Agency. In the draft strategy, three options for managing growth were put forward: concentration, consolidation and dispersal, and the 'business as usual' option where urban growth is less regulated, unguided, and driven by private developer demand.

The core working group of the Greater Christchurch UDS HIA was composed of two public health physicians from the public health unit of the Canterbury DHB and two senior policy analysts from the Christchurch City Council planning and policy team responsible for the strategy. Consultants provided support in some parts of the process (Stevenson et al. 2005).

The specific aims and objectives of the HIA were to:

◆ provide evidence about the links between urban development and health for decision-making

◆ assess the positive and negative health impacts of the UDS and provide recommendations to increase positive and decrease negative impacts

◆ strengthen partnerships between sectors and ensure appropriate participation of the community, including those that are vulnerable due to social exclusion

Table 10.1 New Zealand HIAs underway or completed since 2005

Health determinant	Policy agency	Type of proposal assessed	Number
Urban planning and growth	Regional and local government	Strategy, policy, plan	13*
Transport	Regional and local government	Strategy, programme, project	10
Health services	DHB, local health provider	Policy, programme, plan	7
Water	Central, regional, and local government	Policy, project	3
Alcohol	Local government	Strategy	3
Waste management	Local government	Strategy	1
Housing	Local government	Plan	2
Energy and developments	Central government and industry	Strategy, project	2
Education	High school	Programme	1
Industrial development	Industry	Project	1
Economic factors	Central government	Policy	1
Vandalism	Local government	Strategy	1
Gambling	Local government	Policy	1
Major events	Central government	Programme	1
Total			47

*Most reports and evaluations are available at <http://www.health.govt.nz/our-work/health-impact-assessment/hia-support-unit>.

- ◆ involve Māori in all levels of the HIA process
- ◆ build capacity and knowledge of HIAs in Christchurch and New Zealand (Stevenson et al. 2005).

The HIA included:

- ◆ screening the strategy to determine if it was suitable for an HIA to be conducted
- ◆ scoping the HIA
- ◆ undertaking eight rapid appraisal workshops with a broad range of stakeholders and community members
- ◆ conducting literature reviews

♦ reporting back to workshop participants via the internet and a summary meeting

♦ circulating the HIA report to stakeholders and presenting it to decision makers (Stevenson et al. 2005).

A process and impact evaluation of the HIA found that the HIA had direct impacts on planning and implementation of the final UDS. The evaluation also found the HIA had positive indirect impacts on the understanding of HIA, intersectoral collaboration, and relationships within and between organizations (Mathias and Harris-Roxas 2009).

Analysis of the New Zealand case

A conceptual framework for evaluating HIA is used to critically reflect on the growth and development of HIA in New Zealand (Harris-Roxas and Harris in press). The model, based on context, process, and impacts of HIAs (see Figure 10.1), provides an excellent framework for considering the impacts of HIA.

Context: decision-making and purpose, goals, and values

Context refers to the decision-making context and the purpose, goals, and values of the HIA. The contextual issues discussed above were central to the development of HIA in New Zealand. A key value of New Zealand HIA is equity. Population groups likely to benefit most from a focus on health and wellbeing (such as Māori, Pacific, and low-income peoples) are commonly identified in the screening and scoping stages of HIAs. Care is taken during the HIA appraisal stage to ensure that these communities are included and

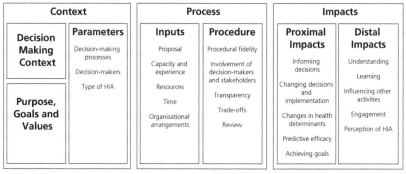

Fig. 10.1 Conceptual framework for evaluating the impact and effectiveness of HIA. Reprinted from Environmental Ben Harris-Roxas and Elizabeth Harris, The Impact and Effectiveness of Health Impact Assessment: A conceptual framework, Environmental Impact Assessment Review, Copyright © 2012, DOI: 10.1016/j.eiar.2012.09.003 with permission from Elsevier.

impacts considered. This commitment to addressing inequalities is, in large part, due to the efforts of successive generations of Māori for equity under the Treaty of Waitangi.

Context: parameters

Parameters set the scene for the HIA. Establishing the parameters for the policy-making process, such as who is making the decision and when, prior to undertaking the HIA has allowed HIA teams to work efficiently. This has ensured that appropriate recommendations are made, in time, to the right people. For example, a number of the New Zealand HIAs have been able to add value to the consultation process with local communities, an important component of the decision-making process for both local government and health (Mathias and Harris-Roxas 2009; McClellan and Signal 2009).

Process: inputs

Inputs refer to the resources available to conduct the HIA. Leadership by the public health community was an essential input in the New Zealand case. The role of the PHAC, particularly its political and administrative independence, put it in a unique position to provide such leadership. It seems likely that HIA would not have advanced as far in New Zealand without PHAC's leadership and support. PHAC developed HIA to the position where it could be picked up by a central government agency. The Ministry of Health established the HIA Support Unit in 2007. Its work continues at the time of writing, but to a lesser extent than when it was first established.

Most DHB public health units have undertaken HIAs. Reasons for this include permission given to them by the Ministry of Health through funding contracts, allocation of staff and funding by DHB management, workforce development resulting in trained staff in all public health units in 2009 (Graves 2010), and the willingness of staff to take a new approach to promoting health. There appears to be increasing acceptance amongst public health staff that HIA is 'business as usual'. Furthermore, several public health units have established dedicated positions to undertake and support HIAs.

Local government has also been a key player in the development of HIA in New Zealand. Several HIAs have been led by local governments and many other HIAs have involved strong collaboration between public health and local government staff. It seems likely that the legislative requirement on local government to consider community wellbeing has been an important motivator for them in adopting HIA. HIA values and processes appear to resonate with some local government staff and politicians. Building support and leadership for HIA in local government is a continuing focus in New Zealand.

The HIA Support Unit has been instrumental in the institutionalization of HIA through awareness raising, provision of technical advice, capacity development, and building an evidence base. A 2009 evaluation of the HIA Support Unit found that as a result of its efforts 'more HIAs have been completed and HIA has greater visibility with policy makers, especially at a regional level' (King et al. 2009). Consultants and academics have also been key players by developing and delivering HIA training programmes, mentoring teams undertaking HIAs, conducting process and impact evaluations, and advising the HIA Support Unit.

A contestable Learning by Doing Fund has provided financial support to nearly half the HIAs undertaken in New Zealand to date. The fund, now ceased, increased the number of HIAs that occurred and may have ensured better quality practice. The learning by doing approach has been dominant in the New Zealand case, with key players deliberately setting out to grow and increase the capacity of the HIA workforce. Success in this is evident in areas such as Hawke's Bay, where the HIA team grew in confidence, skill, and efficiency as they undertook a series of HIAs. Prior to the availability of the fund, most HIAs were funded through existing funding streams in public health units and local government. It is anticipated that the increased HIA capacity in public health units and local government will support continued HIA practice.

Process: procedure

Process refers to how the HIA was conducted. A review was undertaken on ten HIA reports (a subset of the HIAs identified in Table 10.1) (Health, Wellbeing & Equity Impact Assessment Research Unit and Quigley and Watts Ltd 2011). The review concluded that the majority of New Zealand HIAs were good or satisfactory. Several strengths were noted, including the use of a broad definition of health, consideration of the wider determinants of health, and good engagement with stakeholders and representatives of affected communities. Furthermore, decision-makers were often involved in the HIA process, resulting in recommendations that were fit for purpose (Health, Wellbeing & Equity Impact Assessment Research Unit and Quigley and Watts Ltd 2011).

The weaknesses identified included first that 'very few of the HIAs provided a public health profile' and second that very few addressed the size or magnitude of the health impact, despite clear advice about this in the PHAC guidelines. The evaluation authors argued that this was because of lack of local data. Third, 'while equity issues were certainly "on the radar" in the HIAs reviewed, the actual analysis of the distribution of effects was generally weak'. This is a crucial area for improvement in New Zealand, given New

Zealand's values base. Fourth, in some cases HIAs have been undertaken when other approaches may have been more appropriate, possibly due to the availability of HIA funding through the Learning by Doing Fund (Health, Wellbeing & Equity Impact Assessment Research Unit and Quigley and Watts Ltd 2011).

Proximal and distal impacts

Proximal impacts are the things that change most directly as a result of the HIA and distal impacts are more indirect. These impacts are relatively well documented in New Zealand as many of the HIAs have been subject to some form of independent process and impact evaluation. At the proximal level, evaluations suggest that the HIAs contributed positively to the process and content of planned interventions. This ranged from the introduction of new elements into an urban intensification plan, to an amendment of the scope and content of a council bylaw (O'Neill 2011), and the emergence of an entirely new strategy that was adopted and is being implemented (McClellan and Signal 2009).

In relation to distal outcomes, evaluations have demonstrated five key lessons. First, there was a strengthening of intersectoral partnerships. For example, as a result of the UDS HIA, a new position was created for a public health physician in the Christchurch City Council and work commenced on a joint health and local government City Health Plan (Mathias and Harris-Roxas 2009). Second, relationships strengthened between local government, health, and the community. HIA provided an opportunity for voices that have not been well heard in policy-making to have a stronger voice. Again through the UDS HIA, Ngāi Tahu, the local Māori tribe, became more strongly engaged in the UDS process. This was due, in part, to the HIA focus on addressing the needs of Māori and the relationship building of a Māori public health physician on the HIA team (Mathias and Harris-Roxas 2009). Third, awareness was raised in health, local government, the private sector, and the community of the value of focusing on the determinants of health and the need to address health equity. Fourth, an evidence base was built about the health impacts of a range of factors in the New Zealand context (see <http://www.health.govt.nz/our-work/health-impact-assessment/hia-support-unit>). Fifth, HIA strengthened the process of policy-making, resulting in more democratic, consultative, fairer policy that is broader in scope. For example, HIA provided 'a clear voice for Māori policy making', as one leading Māori policy-maker noted (Teresa Wall personal communication): a critical achievement in a nation where Māori life expectancy is about eight years less than that of non-Māori (Blakely et al. 2007).

Conclusion

There is a now a substantial body of work in New Zealand demonstrating the value of HIA at the local level, including how HIA can strengthen health, wellbeing, and equity considerations in strategies, policies, programmes, and plans. This work has included building HIA workforce capacity, increasing the evidence about the impacts of policy on health, and evaluating the benefits of HIA. Furthermore, there has been progress on embedding HIA as 'business as usual' in public health and in some areas of local government. There are many reasons for this progress, including a supportive context of ideas, procedures, and policies; leadership from the public health community, local government, the HIA Support Unit, and consultants and academics; and a strong commitment to addressing inequalities, particularly for Māori.

Progress has slowed since 2009, reflecting reprioritization of resources by successive centre-right governments. For instance, efforts to provide a legal framework for HIA under new public health legislation have stalled and the Learning by Doing Fund is no longer available. Further challenges include how to continue to support and grow HIA, how to strengthen its presence in local government, and, the big challenge for New Zealand, how to get it accepted as 'business as usual' in central government.

Generic learning points

For public health practitioners and policy-makers

◆ Context matters. In New Zealand, HIA emerged from a broader constitutional, legal, and public health context.

◆ It is possible to undertake HIAs that address the broad determinants of health and key values such as equity.

◆ Knowing the parameters of an HIA is important to ensuring that it can be effectively undertaken.

◆ Process matters to the quality and effectiveness of HIA.

◆ Evaluation helps to build the case for HIA and strengthen HIA practice.

◆ HIAs can directly improve the assessed proposal and more distal factors such as inter-sectoral collaboration, relationships with communities, and democratic policy-making.

For educators and researchers

◆ Training aids the translation of theory into practice.

◆ It is possible to promote HIA through learning by doing and embed it in government decision-making.

References

Blakely, T., Tobias, M., Atkinson, J., Yeh, L.-C., and Huang, K. (2007) *Tracking Disparity: Trends in ethnic and socioeconomic inequalities in mortality, 1981–2004*. Wellington: Ministry of Health.

Graves, B. (2010) *Stocktake of Health Impact Assessment Capacity Building Activities in Public Health Units*. Wellington: Ministry of Health.

Harris-Roxas, B. and Harris, E. (in press) The impact and effectiveness of health impact assessment: a conceptual framework. *Environmental Impact Assessment Review*.

Health, Wellbeing & Equity Impact Assessment Research Unit and Quigley and Watts Ltd (2011) *Review of Health Impact Assessments Conducted Under the Ministry of Health Learning by Doing Fund*. Wellington: Ministry of Health.

King, J., Pipi, K., Holmes, R., and Jansen, S. (2009) *Evaluation of the Health Impact Assessment Support Unit*. Wellington: Ministry of Health.

Mahoney, M., Simpson, S., Harris E, Aldrich, R., and Stewart Williams, J. (2004) *Equity focused health impact assessment framework*. Newcastle: The Australasian Collaboration for Health Equity Impact Assessment (ACHEIA), University of Newcastle.

Mathias, K. and Harris-Roxas, B. (2009) Process and impact evaluation of the Greater Christchurch Urban Development Strategy Health Impact Assessment. *BMC Public Health* 9: 97.

McClellan, V. and Signal, L. (2009) *Health Impact Assessment on the Wairoa District Council's Draft Waste Management Activity Plan: The results of a process and impact evaluation*. Wellington: Health, Wellbeing & Equity Impact Assessment Research Unit, University of Otago.

Minister of Health (2000) *The New Zealand Health Strategy*. Wellington: Ministry of Health.

Ministry of Health (2002) *Reducing Inequalities in Health*. Wellington: Ministry of Health.

Ministry of Health (2007) *Whānau Ora Health Impact Assessment*. Wellington: Ministry of Health.

Morgan, R.K. (2008) Institutionalising health impact assessment: the New Zealand experience. *Impact Assessment and Project Appraisal* 26: 2–16.

National Health Committee (1998) *The Social, Cultural and Economic Determinants of Health in New Zealand: action to improve health*. Wellington: National Health Committee.

O'Neill, E. (2011) *Evaluation Report for the Central Dunedin Speed Restriction Health Impact Assessment*. Dunedin: Dunedin City Council.

Public Health Advisory Committee (2004) *A Guide to Health Impact Assessment: a policy tool for New Zealand*. Wellington: Public Health Advisory Committee.

Quigley, R. and Burt, S. (2006) Assessing the health and wellbeing impacts of urban planning in Avondale: a New Zealand case study. *Social Policy Journal of New Zealand* 29: 165–175.

Stevenson, A., Banwell, K. and Pink, R. (2005) *A Health Impact Assessment of the Greater Christchurch Urban Development Strategy*. Christchurch: Canterbury District Health Board.

Urban Development Forum (2004) *Urban Development Forum: Greater Christchurch Urban Development Strategy—So many options, which will you choose?* Christchurch: Christchurch City Council.

Chapter 11

A decade of health impact assessment development in Thailand: from cases to constitution

Decharut Sukkumnoed

Introduction

This chapter firstly provides the historical development and philosophical basis of health impact assessment (HIA) development in Thailand since 2000, through the facilitation of the Health System Reform Office (HSRO). Then, the legislative process of HIA from 2000 to 2007 is described, which hopefully can provide a lesson learned for other countries. After that, the present HIA institutional mechanism and implementation in Thailand is explained, before critical reflection on an existing HIA system in Thailand is presented. At the end of the chapter, the conclusion and generic learning points from HIA development in Thailand are outlined.

Background

The concepts of healthy public policy (HPP) and HIA were initially introduced to Thai society during the process of the national health system reform, which commenced in 2000. This reform provides important opportunities and processes for several changes in Thai society, including the expansion and deep-rooting of HPP and HIA.

Combined with drastic changes in social and political conditions during the 1980s and 1990s, the national health system was increasingly forced to reform. A climax was reached in 1997 when the new Thai constitution was adopted and implemented, which was heavily influenced by civil society. Under this constitutional reform, health became a part of human rights—not just public welfare. Consequently, the government was required to provide public health services of the same standard to all population groups. Concurrently, all development programmes and projects that had adverse impacts on health are now required to conduct impact assessment (IA) with a public scrutiny process. The civic roles in policy formulations and public decision-making, as well as in their implementation, had been asserted in the Thai constitution (Phoolcharoen 2004).

The drafting process of the National Health Act

The National HSRO, an ad hoc organization created under the Health Systems Research Institute (HSRI), functioning as the secretarial division of the National Health System Reform Committee, was established in 2000 by the Prime Minister's Office Regulation on National Health System Reform.

As a secretarial body, HSRO had coordinated with all sectors throughout the country to take part in the conceptualization and the formulation of the National Health Act, which was to be a health statute in Thai society. The HSRO also used this process as a learning mechanism for Thai people towards the reform of their health behaviours and modes of thinking in order to move from 'health repair' to 'health promotion'.

The tangible outcome of the reform was to develop the National Health Act as a constitutional framework of the national health system. However, unlike other legislation in Thailand, the reform aimed to use a drafting process as an opportunity for mutual learning in Thai society.

The process was started from the national level and then through six regional seminars on the topic 'The Desirable Health System in Thailand' in 2000. The results of these seminars were collated and later informed the background paper for developing the framework of health system reform. In January 2001, the principle framework for national health system reform was developed and was followed by a public hearing and feedback process. Around 35,000 people from more than 1800 organizations joined the public hearings held in every province of the country. The framework, feedback process, and other ideas were discussed and summarized in the first National Health Assembly in September 2001 (Phoolcharoen 2004).

Health as wellbeing

Through this reform process, several new ideas in the health system were introduced, demonstrated, deliberatively discussed, and iteratively developed, which have led to significant changes in the dimensions of health within Thai society.

The new dimensions emerge from the definition of health. In the draft, health was defined as 'the complete status holistically interrelated in the physical, mental, social, and spiritual balances' (National Health System Reform

Committee 2002: 2), therefore health is no longer connected to the issue of ill-ness. It becomes the issue of complete wellbeing, both for individuals and the whole society, and both in physical and more social and spiritual senses.

Following on from this new definition of health, health systems are now referred to as 'all of the interconnected management that enhance healthiness and factors relevant to health aspects, such as individual factors; economic, social, political, educational, legal, religious, cultural and traditional factors; scientific and technology factors; as well as the factors on public health and public health service' (National Health System Reform Committee 2002: 2). In other words, the health system is moving beyond the previously familiar 'health sector'.

The draft also asserts the right of people to participate, with the state and the community, in generating the environmental conditions that are appropriate, balanced, safe, quality-assured, and which meet the standard of continuous normal living with good health. Therefore, the new health system aims to cre-ate health for all and facilitates all sectoral participation to enhance health promotion (National Health System Reform Committee 2002).

HIA development in Thailand

The issues of HPP and HIA were raised firstly during the national seminar on 'The Desirable Health System in Thailand' in 2000 and echoed during the public hearings at the provincial level in 2001. This issue has become more important for Thai society, mainly because of the increasing trend of health risks from environmental hazards such as air pollution, pesticide contamina-tions, improper waste treatments, and so on, as well as the evidence and con-cerns of health impacts from development projects such as large dams, power plants, trans-national gas pipelines, highways, and so on.

After this was raised in the reform process, the HSRI set up the academic review process in 2001, which, consequently, reinforced the concept of HPP, as introduced in the Ottawa Charter (1986). The notion of HPP received a good public response in combating problems faced by Thai society and was put into the national health system reform framework (Phoolcharoen et al. 2003).

Later, in 2001, the issue of HPP became the first topic of discussion in the first National Health Assembly, showing its relevancy and importance in the Thai health reform context. In the assembly discussion, two HIAs conducted on the industrial development project and agricultural policy were presented, showing clear negative health impacts from these well-known government initiatives. As a result of the first assembly, the concepts of HPP and HIA were included in the first draft of the National Health Act, paving the way for HSRI to develop a research programme on HPP and HIA that started in

2002, in order to support further development in HPP and HIA in Thailand (Phoolcharoen et al. 2003).

The draft stresses that the expected health system will have guidelines and measures to establish HPP and the process for HIA from the public policy, aimed at joint learning of all sectors in society. Furthermore, the draft also asserts the right of Thai people to participate in using the assessment outputs and making decisions on policy implementation and crucial projects that may have an impact on health (National Health System Reform Committee 2002).

From 2002, the HIA guidelines and capacity-strengthening activities were carried out for both academics and active citizens. Under the HSRI research programme, over 50 HIA case studies were conducted on several policy issues, at both national and local levels. Although all the cases aimed at desirable policy changes, only some of them were able to influence this, highlighting the importance of policy contexts in HPP developments.

HIA in the legislative process

In Thailand, the constitution allows Thai people to collectively submit a bill to parliament. The recommendations and academic syntheses were included in the content of the National Health Bill, which was then taken to the public consultation process through all provincial health assemblies. The last consultation was organized in August 2002 in the national health assembly, and the Bill was reviewed in September 2002. This law was generally known as 'the people issue of the Health Act' and included seven sections referring to HIA (National Health System Reform Committee 2002).

HSRO submitted the Bill to the Government, and the Council of State was then assigned to review and amend many sections. The Bill was, therefore, called 'the Government's issue'. Moreover, only two sections referring to HIA remained after the amendment. The Bill was firstly approved with the consensus of the House of Representatives in December 2005 (Jindawattana 2010). However, a political crisis in 2006, which led to the coup d'etat on 19 September 2006, brought the National Health Bill back to the beginning of its legislative process.

Shortly after the establishment of the National Legislative Assembly, the National Health Bill was submitted to it. The amendment commission was established to review the Bill with the participation of the people representatives of the previous Health Assemblies. With the full support from these commissioners, the rights and participation of the citizens in HIA are restored in Sections 10 and 11 in the final National Health Bill (see Box 11.1).

Box 11.1 Extracts from the National Health Act B.E.2550 (2007)

Section 10 In the case where there exists an incident affecting public health, a State agency having information relating to such incident shall expeditiously disclose such information and the protection thereof to the public.

Section 11 An individual or group of people has the right to request for estimation or participating in the estimation of impact on health resulting from a public policy.

An individual or group of people shall have access to information, explanation and underlying reason prior to a permission or performance of a programme or activity which may affect his or her health or the health of a community, and shall have the right to express his or her opinion on such matter.

Section 25 (5) National Health Commission (NHC) shall have powers and duties to prescribe rules and procedure on following up and evaluation in respect of national health system and the impact on health resulting from public policies, both in the levels of policy making and implementation.

Source: Extracts reproduced from National Health Commission Office (2008) National Health Act BE.2550 (2007). Bangkok: National Health Commission Office. copyright © 2008.

Finally, on 4 January 2007, the National Legislative Assembly approved the National Health Bill. As mentioned earlier, this time the rights and participation of the citizens in HIA are restored in Sections 10 and 11, while the prescription of HIA criteria and methods is stated in Section 25(5) (Jindawattana 2010).

The National Health Act B.E.2550 (2007) (see Box 11.1) is one of a few laws in Thailand that have the most extensive people participation process in the history of Thailand. It is the first Act that includes several sections on HIA. The Act covers the right, responsibilities, and functions for health and health securities (National Health Commission Office 2008).

Moving into the constitution

After the success in implementing the HIA National Health Act, HIA was discussed in the drafting process of the new constitution. The National Legislative Assembly, which passed the National Health Act, also suggested adding HIA in the decision process of projects and activities that may be harmful to the health of Thai people. Later, HIA was added to the draft of the national constitution and was passed through the first national referendum in August 2007. Finally, since August 2007, HIA has been acknowledged in the national constitution. The Constitution of the Kingdom of Thailand BE.2550 (2007) in section 67 stipulates that (Royal Thai Parliament 2007):

> 'Any project or activity which may seriously affect a community's environmental quality, its natural resources **or its people's health**, is prohibited unless (a) **these environmental and health impacts are studied and assessed** (b) a public hearing process is undertaken to obtain the opinions of people and stakeholders and (c) independent organization formed by representatives of non-governmental organizations and higher education institutes provides opinions and comments, prior to the implementation of such a project or activity...' [chapter author's emphasis]

Present HIA mechanisms in Thailand

Based on both the National Constitution and the National Health Act, HIA in Thailand has been applied in four main ways.

Firstly, as mentioned earlier, according to the Constitution, all possible harmful projects require the conduct of HIA in their decision-making processes. In the HIA process, regarding possible harmful projects, local people and the public can participate meaningfully in public scoping and public review. According to the constitution, each HIA report must be reviewed by the independent organization in order to ensure the quality of the HIA process and report.

Secondly, any governmental organizations may apply HIA in the policy and planning development. Therefore, in addition to the project level, HIA can also be applied at the policy and programme levels, such as for nuclear/energy power development planning, for mining development strategy, or for regional development policy. The National Health Commission Office must coordinate with, and support, the relevant organization to conduct HIA in their planning process and facilitate for public participation in the HIA process.

Thirdly, any local people who may be concerned about the impacts of a specific policy on their health also have the right to request for an HIA to be considered in order to ensure that the policy would not lead to negative health impacts. In this case, the National Health Commission Office would facilitate the HIA process, especially the coordination between local people, policy-makers, and relevant organizations in conducting HIA and in applying HIA to the policy-making process.

In Thailand, after the completion of a project or activity where health impacts have occurred, people can still request a retrospective HIA for such a project or activity, as stipulated by the National Health Act. Although, in principle, HIA should be used prospectively, the retrospective HIA can also be very useful for policy evaluation. As a result, the owners of a project or activity may have to undertake measures to eliminate the impact.

Lastly, local governments, the public, and other organizations can apply HIA as a social learning process to solve their own problems or to plan for their better future health. In this case, HIA can be done locally without any law requirement and can communicate with National Health Commission Office for technical support and for an exchange of ideas and information.

To coordinate the overall development of HIA in Thailand the National Health Commission has established the National HIA Commission. Moreover, an HIA Co-ordination Centre has been set up by the National Health Commission Office to facilitate all these HIA implementations.

Critical reflection towards practical solutions

In reality, the implementation of HIA in Thailand has not always run smoothly. In the beginning HIA was regarded as a social learning process in order to come up with the best policy, the so-called HPP, that would be beneficial to the Thai people's health and wellbeing. The effort was successful to a certain degree but locally affected people still hoped that HIA would have more influential power on the government's decisions.

Nevertheless, when the HIA status was 'incorporated' into the 'government's decision-making process' as was expected by the people, questions still remained. Even though section 67 of the constitution has been carried out for almost two years, the private sector still asks for tangible standards and practices for HIA to facilitate the approval process.

Concurrently, local people who live in the Mab Ta Put industrial area, the largest industrial estate in the eastern coast of Thailand, want their concerns and needs to preserve their livelihoods to be included and analysed in HIA as well as to be accepted by other parts of the society, whilst the government and some people in the private sector regard them as 'emotional', not providing reliable information to be used in HIA.

HIA in the Thai constitution remains stuck in the dilemma between a governmental approval process and as a social learning process. This dilemma led the National Health Commission Office to organize the critical reflection workshops for further HIA development in the next five years in 2010 and 2011, with participants from four parties, namely governmental, private, locally affected people, and academic sectors. The results of the workshop are quite critical and interesting, as discussed in the following sections (National Health Commission Office 2010; Sukkumnoed 2011).

Moving upstream of the development process

The lesson from HIAs conducted on project developments has been that HIA should be conducted earlier, at the strategic planning stages. This would enable better engagement throughout the conceptual and strategic development of projects and plans, rather than solely at the end-stage of project development when approval is required, which, in several cases, leads to conflict between proponents and opponents of the projects.

If we want to maintain the spirit of deliberative decision-making within society, HIA must be used as a planning and decision-making tool at the very beginning of project development. Even though each group may have different expectations and ideas about the project development, as long as they have not decided on their standpoints or specific ideas of the project, then there is still some room for social learning and mutual understanding instead of arguments and conflicts where everybody only focuses on the benefits or problems that they desire to receive from the project.

◆ Providing alternative policy options

Although moving towards the upstream in the development process would provide a broader opportunity to share and learn within society, this opportunity cannot be effectively linked to policy solutions until the new strategic policy options are presented, discussed, and analysed through the HIA process. This is because, without policy options, it is quite difficult for Thai society to exchange, learn, and making decisions together. HIA should therefore not only focus on comments and critiques of a specific government policy but also stimulate and accumulate new ideas and initiatives from different stakeholders within the society.

◆ Linking to other aspects of sustainable development

Another major problem for HIA implementation in Thailand is how to link all health determinants into HIA and into the government's decision-making process, especially in the case of the social determinants of health. Since the accuracy of data within the scope of social determinants is often criticized, HIA conducted in Thailand, especially after the 2007 constitution, has mostly focused on the physical and biological environmental aspects rather than psychological, social, or spiritual aspects, as stressed in the National Health Act.

This imbalance, apart from affecting the integrity of HIA, also reduces the importance of local people's voices. As a consequence, the impacts caused by changes of social determinants of health cannot be measured or converted into usable data. Inevitably, this kind of impact is often excluded from HIA or even if it is included, it does not add much weight to the government's decision.

The challenge of HIA therefore is how to develop an HIA scheme that reflects changes in social and spiritual health dimensions. Recent developments in the last two to three years, including the survey of happiness levels of Thai people and the survey of progress indicators all over the country are important steps for the development of databases and tools for HIA to link with and utilize.

◆ **HIA co-ownership**

Last but not least, it is necessary for HIA in the near future to be designed in a way that all sectors, especially local people who will be impacted upon(both positively and negatively), can participate as the owners of the assessment in order to ensure that the assessment really is a social learning process. Consequently, we must be careful when developing tools and databases not to lessen the sense of ownership of HIA in both the community and other sectors. Tools should only support communication and sharing of information and opinions amongst various parties rather than be used as the sole answer in the decision-making process.

Building a system that would enable everybody to work together for HIA, for example database developers, future scenario simulators, impacted people, official decision-makers, and other groups, is a real challenge for Thai society. This is a cultural challenge for creating IA and a decision-making process that is mutually owned by various parties instead of the privately owned assessment or state-centered approach that has been used in the past.

Conclusion

Within just one decade, HIA development in Thailand has journeyed from being an initial idea in 2000, to becoming part of an overall institutional framework. It must be remembered, however, that focusing on the institutional infrastructure cannot lead to the full development of HIA as a desirable social learning. HIA in Thailand has moved from conferences and case studies towards the constitution. In this aspect, HIA can work as a process and tool for Thai people to protect their rights and, at the same time, for Thai policymakers to share with all stakeholders.

Generic learning points

For public health practitioners and policy-makers

◆ Through encouraging and facilitating local people to take part in the policy process with more reliable evidence and effective recommendations, HIA can be seen as a civic empowerment process.

◆ HIA can be a useful tool for deliberative policy analysis, which is critical and essential for conflict resolution in policy process.

For educators and researchers

◆ HIA requires both institutional framework and analytical framework developments.

◆ HIA co-ownership is critical for the success of HIA implementation. It can be mainly done through capacity strengthening of all stakeholders and the development of an appropriate analytical framework.

You can learn more about HIA development in Thailand through the HIA Co-ordination Centre (<http://www.thia.in.th/>).

Bibliography

Jindawattana, A. (2010) *HIA: Catalyst or Inhibitor for Development in Thailand.* [in Thai] Bangkok: National Health Commission Office.

National Health Commission Office (2008) National Health Act BE.2550 (2007). Bangkok: National Health Commission Office.

National Health Commission Office (2010) *HIA in Thailand in the Next Five Years.* [in Thai] Bangkok: National Health Commission Office.

National Health System Reform Committee (2002) *The Draft Law of National Health as a Thais' Health Constitution,* revised edition. Bangkok: Health System Reform Office.

Phoolcharoen, W. (2004) *Quantum Leap: The Reform of Thailand's Health System.* Bangkok: Health Systems Research Institute.

Phoolcharoen, W., Sukkumnoed, D., and Kessomboon, P. (2003) Development of health impact assessment in thailand: recent experiences and challenges. *Bulletin of the World Health Organization* 81 (6): 465–467.

Royal Thai Parliament (2007) *The Constitution of Kingdom of Thailand B.E. 2550 (2007)* Bangkok: Royal Thai Parliament.

Sukkumnoed, D. (2011) *HIA 2.0: The New Challenge for Thai Society.* Bangkok: Healthy Public Policy Foundation.

(2008) *National Health Act BE.2550 (2007).* Bangkok: National Health Commission Office. copyright © 2008.

Chapter 12

From instrument towards a health in all policies programme for inter-sectoral decision support: health impact assessment in The Netherlands

Marleen Bekker, Mieke Steenbakkers, Ilse Storm, and Maria Jansen

Introduction

In The Netherlands, as in many countries worldwide, local governments are by national law responsible for local integrated public health policy. This approach has also been cited as health in all policies (HiAP). A precondition to realize HiAP is inter-sectoral collaboration between a municipality's policy sectors and subsequently with external private or public organizations. So far, there is limited knowledge either on how to organize cross-sectoral partnerships at the local level or the impact of inter-sectoral collaboration between policy sectors and integrated policy proposals. The health impact assessment (HIA) approach provides an opportunity to discuss the health impacts of measures taken by non-health policy sectors and therefore to build up cross-sectoral cooperation.

We will briefly recall the conclusions of two major evaluations of HIA and integrated health policies in The Netherlands published in 2007. We then turn to answer the central question: How are integrated health policies, either using HIA or not, developed in 2010, and how can we use insights in the processes and outcomes to provide further guidance in establishing these policies? Then we will describe which changes have taken place since, first describing the national policy context, followed by the results of two studies of local inter-sectoral collaboration and integrated health policies published in 2010. Given these case studies, this chapter focuses on the public health format of HIA rather than the environmental format. After summarizing the difficulties and dilemmas that persist at the local level, we will propose a programmatic approach towards HiAP, in which HIA can be embedded for more sustainable impact.

Background

In The Netherlands, HIA was introduced in the national policy memorandum *Healthy and Sound* (Gezond en wel) in 1995. Evaluation research on the policy impact of national and local HIAs in 2007 indicated that HIA had not been very effective in The Netherlands. On the one hand, the design of HIA, emphasizing scientific soundness at the expense of stakeholder consideration, obstructed rather than facilitated the integration of the health aspect in public policy (Bekker 2007). On the other hand, HIA and HiAP proposals were often opposed by the higher civil servants within the public health sector, who were protecting their minister from political harm. Bekker concluded that the scientifically objective presentation of health impacts in the investigated Dutch HIAs did not match the normative, value-ridden policy process. Alternatively, building a consensus among the HIA researchers and policy stakeholders involved might neutralize the political sensitivities concerning the collision of health and non-health policy priorities, and the HIA as a policy evaluation instrument.

Additionally, in a study of the interactions between researchers, policy-makers, and public health professionals at the municipal level, Jansen concluded that collaborations often stumbled at the organizational middle-management level because of a lack of leadership, support, and available means (Jansen et al. 2008). Jansen proposed a sustained dialogue between the actors and stakeholders from the policy sectors and executive organizations involved in order to improve the interconnections between the sectors. Interactions between stakeholders at the strategic, managerial, and operational levels would facilitate knowledge sharing and subsequent improvements in HiAP.

Before we dive into a number of case studies of integrated health policies in 2010, we first describe which contextual policy changes have taken place, possibly providing new incentives for HiAP.

Recent policy developments

On the one hand, the national government since 2007 has implemented a number of policy measures that may reduce barriers to HiAP. First of all, national government is increasingly decentralizing health and welfare tasks to local governments. Nowadays, municipalities are responsible for the implementation of the Dutch Public Health Act as well as for the Social Support Act, which aims at the social participation of all citizens. Since 2008, municipalities have also been responsible for the Youth and Family Centres, which provide integrated preventive care and support to families and youngsters. Additionally, youth social support will be decentralized from 2014 onwards. Finally, the recent national Public Health memorandum states that public–private collaboration might give more room for HiAP and integration of local memoranda. It advocates a shared responsibility of local government, industries, private companies, social institutes, the education sector, and care providers, whereas formerly it was a responsibility of local governments only. At the national level, the Healthy Living Centre has been established to carry out work on HiAP (e.g. the *Healthy City Guide*).

On the other hand, instruments such as HIA, determinant policy screening (DPS), and the quick scan (QS) are not legally required in the development of HiAP. In Dutch national policy, only environmental impact assessment (EIA) and strategic environmental assessment (SEA) are legally required, which provide some room for the consideration of health aspects of environmental impacts. Additionally, the Ministry pays lip service to the use of the public health HIA (including all health determinants) at the local level. Nevertheless, there have been no formal policy incentives to introduce public health HIAs since around 2003.

HiAP in 2010

Although the number of municipalities that address HiAP in their local health policy document has risen to 76%, only 15% of these documents describe supporting methods for HiAP such as HIA, DPS, or QS. Two recent studies analyse the Dutch local practices and explore opportunities with regard to inter-sectoral collaboration between municipality's policy sectors and subsequently with external private or public organizations (as an important prerequisite for HiAP).

Study 1: HiAP in Dutch municipalities (Storm et al. 2010)

This study was carried out by the National Institute for Public Health and the Environment and was assigned by the Ministry of Health, Welfare and Sports to support municipalities that want to establish HiAP. It included 16 municipalities where HiAP to some extent had been developed. The aim was to clarify processes which play a role with regard to the development and implementation of such a policy to reduce health inequalities.

Methods

Based on a survey, in-depth interviews, and a work conference, experiences of local policy officers at the operational level from inside and outside the public health sector are explicated. The analysis addresses both content of policies, i.e. activities, as well as the collaboration process between policy officers.

Results

In general, the encountered activities are related to integral projects rather than integrated policies. Moreover, the activities focus on lifestyle rather than the physical environmental component of health, consisting of health-promoting interventions rather than health-protecting measures. With regard to the reduction of health inequalities, sectors and parties seem to prefer to collaborate on projects focusing on themes such as being overweight, alcohol abuse, and psycho-social problems.

Increasingly, municipalities collaborate in the development and implementation of health programmes, e.g. Healthy School and Healthy City, or social programmes, e.g. an action plan for a deprived neighbourhood. Often, such programmes are an effective means to promote collaboration between different parties. These more comprehensive programmes are supported by municipalities, partly sponsored by the national government, and monitored on both inter-sectoral linkages and results.

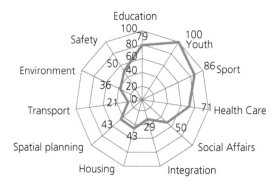

Percentage health policy officers

Health policy officers

Fig. 12.1 Collaboration between health policy officers and non-health policy officers to reduce health inequalities.

In general, the public health sector primarily collaborates with social sectors, i.e. youth, education, sport, and social affairs, and less with physical environment ones, i.e. spatial planning, housing, and environments (see Figure 12.1). The health sector would like to collaborate more with the physical sectors because health inequalities are closely related to poor living and environmental conditions.

Analysing the process, mutual acquaintance seems to be a starting point for collaboration. A learning process is considered a precondition for expressing and adjusting mutual expectations. To date, agreements on collaboration differ by municipality (for instance who is in control and what method is being followed). Municipalities also seldom use HIA to discuss the health impact of measures taken by non-health policy sectors. Just one out of the 16 municipalities in this study executed the specific HIA City and Environment (an environmental health focused format of HIA), and none of the 16 carried out the general HIA. Because of the diversity of the municipalities there is no uniform approach in which HIAP was developed and implemented. Determining factors for collaboration are priorities, themes, the used methods, the culture, i.e. experience, and the scale of the municipalities involved. Opportunities exist mainly where the importance of inter-sectoral collaboration is acknowledged on all hierarchic levels of the municipality.

Conclusions

Storm et al. conclude that although both health and other local departments develop numerous health-relevant activities, these are not well integrated. The manner and the degree in which organizations both outside and inside the public health sector collaborate to address the problem of health inequalities differs per municipality. On the local level, there are potential improvement points identified to broaden and intensify collaboration among the various sectors, including alignment of health with local priorities, enhancing parallel interests, the improvement of alignment with physical sectors, identification of keyholders and clarifying roles, the establishment of political and administrative support, and coherence of objectives and methods.

Study 2: Coaching municipalities in setting up inter-sectoral policies (Steenbakkers et al. 2012)

In South Limburg a more cooperative HIA model through knowledge sharing and dialogue was developed, involving operational, managerial, and strategic levels of the organizational stakeholders in integrated policy efforts. The regional Public Health Service (PHS) together with the National Institute on

Health Promotion and Disease Prevention (NIHPDP) developed a coaching programme for stakeholders in the region to collaboratively find ways to develop HiAP, using obesity as an example. The coaching programme lasted 30 months (from May 2007 until November 2009).

The coaching programme

The coaching programme distinguished between stakeholders at the strategic, managerial, and operational levels of the organizations involved. At the strategic level, three regional conferences were held with municipal councillors with a public health portfolio, addressing the need for agenda setting, showing visible commitment and leadership, and creating resources for inter-sectoral collaboration on the issue of obesity.

At the managerial level, the managers were only informed by the municipal councillors and civil servants, they were not actively involved. In most municipalities, the policy-making capacity of public health is very small (on average 8 hours a week, range 4–32). Managers had to agree to allow the public health civil servant a minimal extra time investment of two hours per week.

At the operational level, a master class for civil servants and PHS professionals on promoting inter-sectoral collaboration was held. The application of policy instruments, e.g. HIA, DPS, and QS, was suggested. Active learning was stimulated by the formation of a trio of the public health civil servant from the municipality, the PHS professional, and the health promoter of the NIHPDP. In seven meetings experts trained skills and reflected on the local activities of the trios. The trios were expected to build HiAP plans that would be agreed on in local government and would therefore be ready for implementation.

Methods

Based on survey analysis before and after the coaching programme (9 coached municipalities were compared to 23 non-coached municipalities), log book registries, and in-depth interviews with municipal managers public health, outcomes were scored depending on the stage of HiAP proposals (range 0–5, no HiAP to ready for implementation of HiAP).

Results

Six of the nine coached municipalities showed concrete outcomes of HiAP. Two municipalities withdrew from participation prematurely (score 0) and one could not achieve any policy result (score 1). In three municipalities the issue of health promotion was included in policy documents but the proposal was still in the preparation stage (score 2). One municipality included a health check for obesity in spatial planning and environmental policy proposals that was ready for decision (score 3). In one municipality, a new policy procedure was accepted stating that the public health civil servant should participate in multi-sectoral consultations about environmental policy proposals (score 4). Finally, one municipality expanded an existing evidenced-based HiAP intervention for people with financial problems.

The higher the number of activities and stakeholders' involvement registered in the log book, the higher the outcome score for the stage of HiAP (see Figure 12.2). Despite specific attention during the coaching process, none of the coached municipalities used the HIA, DPS, or QS instruments.

The main differences in pre- and post test measurements were:

1. a decrease in the political priority awarded to HiAP among public health councillors
2. a decrease in managerial support
3. no changes in attitude and self-efficacy among public health civil servants
4. an increase in the number of civil servants outside the public health sector that did not perceive any link with the obesity problem.

These unexpected disappointing effects are still not fully explained. The in-depth interviews with municipal managers revealed that in principle they supported HiAP as 'nobody can be against it'. They were prepared to invest

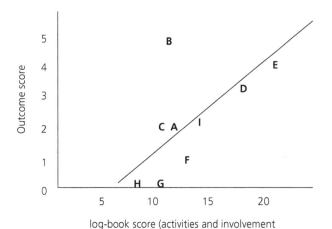

Fig. 12.2 Results of coached municipalities (N = 9: A t/m I). Outcome score related to the log-book score with a maximum of 24 counting activities and involvement during the coaching programme on strategic (max. subscore 8), managerial (max. subscore 7), and operational level (max subscore 9).

in time and personnel if the merits of collaboration with other policy sectors were made clear. Apparently, neither the trio coaching the municipalities nor the regional PHS has so far been able to convince managers of the merits of inter-sectoral collaboration. Additionally, which may or may not be related, two of the nine municipal councillors with public health in their portfolio and six of the nine public health civil servants changed their positions during the coaching programme.

Conclusions

The coaching programme gave a small positive contribution to the implementation of HiAP targeting obesity, as we could see in three out of the nine coached municipalities. But at the strategic and managerial level, political priority and managerial support decreased. The results further showed that more support of the stakeholders at each system level was related to further development of HiAP proposals. Stakeholders at the managerial level were difficult to involve and, in the eyes of coached civil servants, the support for HiAP decreased.

The coaching programme may have insufficiently focused on horizontally organized managerial support, i.e. the inter-sectoral relations between health and non-health policy sectors. Without managerial support, professionals at the operational level have no authority to change their practices, even if they themselves should prefer to work more horizontally, i.e. with other policy sectors, therefore managerial support is essential for innovations. Adjustment of the coaching programme is needed towards active involvement of managers. Finally, professional discontinuity, especially at the operational level, made it difficult to raise knowledge and skills within the municipality.

Persisting difficulties and dilemmas in 2010

From both studies we may conclude that the persistent failure of incentives to apply instruments for HiAP is still a black box. We may only presume that explanations consist of a complex interplay of local factors concerning knowledge, skills, interpersonal relationships, managerial support, and continuity of staffing.

According to the Dutch Inspectorate, Dutch municipalities are confronted with inadequately and insufficiently developed expertise. Municipalities are not aware of the positive effects that health might have on the local economy and residents' participation. Despite some incentives The Netherlands lack a formally established rule of law for HiAP, such as exists in the UK, Finland, or Sweden. Nevertheless, given the history of HiAP, we do not expect sufficient political support for such a rule of law. The conclusions of the 2007 evaluation are still valid: the Dutch conditions for, and applications of, HIA are inadequate in actively engaging all relevant stakeholders, including middle managers, for integrated health policies.

How could these persisting difficulties and dilemmas be more effectively met in the future?

Ideas and practical solutions

Based on the studies described, we have a number of recommendations to improve the opportunities for inter-sectoral collaboration and HiAP in The Netherlands. Depending on the context for application, these may be more, or less, helpful in other countries.

- Develop a programmatic approach around:
  - HIA or other initiatives as embedded and long-term strategies that are effectively linked to budget and decision-making cycles, performance indicators, and allocated responsibilities to municipal departments, managers, and servants
  - building and sustaining a continuous dialogue to identify and sustain parallel interests
  - actively engaging the middle manager of stakeholder organizations to ensure both vertical connections within their own policy sector and horizontal connections with other local policies sectors and external partners
  - clarifying roles: the identified roles in the process of building HiAP (policy entrepreneur, expert, knowledge broker, process manager) can be explored and elaborated in unorthodox training settings where participants actually practice the necessary skills to understand and manage complex conditions (i.e. in gaming or responsive simulations of the process).

- Expand the toolbox for decision-support by:
  - applying the process assessment and design tools that provide a feasibility diagnosis and guidelines for process-oriented action
  - making costs, benefits, and risks transparent to help in reducing uncertainty and managing the investment risks of strategic alliances by the stakeholder organizations that are needed to support and execute the programme (integrated impact assessment)
  - adopting the technique of policy scenarios: visualizing and comparing the various policy options, feasibility, and possible effects may help in reducing uncertainty and managing policy risks.

- Create national policy support and incentives by:
  - network facilitation, making knowledge accessible, and creating a sense of urgency.

Conclusions

Since 2007, the legal incentives for developing HiAP have been the Public Health Act and the Social Support Act. Many municipalities develop numerous activities without being conscious that these actually enhance (or damage) public health. Integrating these activities with public health policies therefore might be easier than is often perceived. Nevertheless, the role of middle managers in prioritizing activities and means for inter-sectoral collaboration and integrated policies should be further investigated. Moreover, the available policy integration tools, such as HIA or DPS, are neither legally required nor known or considered practicable by civil servants.

Opportunities for inter-sectoral collaboration are enhanced by a coaching programme, but Steenbakkers et al. found that middle managers show the least support for this. Major bottlenecks remain the lack of knowledge, competences, and administrative and professional continuity. Moreover, in 16 municipalities where integrated policies to some extent were developed, Storm et al. conclude that although both health and other local departments develop numerous activities, these are not well integrated.

From the 2007 and 2010 evaluation studies we conclude that an infrastructure is needed to embed the current standalone initiatives for HIA in the organization of the regional Public Health Services. The PHSs should position themselves as the regional knowledge centres, providing municipalities with the expertise and continuity needed. Such a programme should link the current ad hoc projects to the operational processes and most importantly to the municipal budget and control cycles. In this way such a programme may also facilitate middle manager engagement, as it establishes points of accountability in the control cycle. The programme allows for a more cohesive, longer-term strategy. The toolbox may be expanded with decision-support tools such as financial outcome analyses and policy scenario-building.

Neither of these recommendations ensures that inter-sectoral collaborations and integrated policies will increase. In the absence of national rules of law and local leadership, they do, however, make local governance of inter-sectoral collaborations and integrated policies more tangible and manageable.

Generic learning points

For public health practitioners and policy-makers

- ◆ Create more political and administrative support at the managerial and strategic municipal levels.
- ◆ Engage process managers and knowledge brokers besides the political entrepreneur and practitioner.
- ◆ Align health priorities with local political priorities such as social participation and social cohesion.
- ◆ Align health priorities with urban development or spatial planning priorities.

For educators and researchers

- ◆ Pay specific attention to the institutional and political contexts in which HIA is practised and the ways in which these can be effectively dealt with. This implies a combination of training cognitive competences for programme management and social skills involving negotiation, process management, and conflict management.

References

Bekker, M.P.M. (2007) *The Politics of Healthy Policies. Redesigning Health Impact Assessment to integrate health in public policy*. PhD thesis. Erasmus University Rotterdam. Delft: Eburon.

Jansen, M.W.J., De Vries, N.K., Kok, G., and Van Oers, H.A.M. (2008) Collaboration between practice, policy and research in local public health in The Netherlands. *Health Policy* 86: 295–307.

Storm, I., Savelkoul, M., Busch, M.C.M., Maas, J., and Schuit, A.J. (2010). Intersectoral collaboration in tackling health inequalities. A study of sixteen municipalities in the Netherlands (in Dutch). Bilthoven: RIVM.

Steenbakkers, M., Jansen, M., Maarse, H., and de Vries, N. (2012) Challenging Health in All Policies, an action research study in Dutch municipalities. *Health Policy* 105: 288–295.

Chapter 13

Health in impact assessment and emerging challenges in India

Ben Cave, Urmila Jha-Thakur, Mala Rao,
Pawan Labhasetwar, and Thomas B. Fischer

Introduction

India is in the process of demographic, economic, epidemiological, and cli-
matic transition and faces challenges to the state of her public's health. It is
clearly important that public policy addresses and attempts to manage this
change while also seeking to achieve sustainability, equitable development,
and continuous improvement of the quality of life, health, and wellbeing of the
whole population. Indeed, Article 47 of the Constitution of India (Government
of India 2011) establishes the duty of the State to raise the level of nutrition and
the standard of living, and to improve public health. Recent UN publications
make a persuasive case for the contribution that the public health workforce
can make at different policy levels (Commission on the Social Determinants
of Health 2008; WHO and United Nations Human Settlements Programme
2010). We ask whether equipping this workforce with appropriate skills and
competence can help shape responses to these challenges. Can a public health
perspective inform and contribute to the inclusive and sustainable growth to
which the Government of India aspires, and which has the support of organizations such as the multilateral lender, the Asian development Bank (ADB)
(ADB 2012)?

Health impact assessment (HIA) is a systematic process by which to identify the potential health effects of policies, plans, programmes, and projects
whether they be inside or outside the health sector. HIA also identifies strategies for managing any effects that are identified (Quigley et al. 2006) and it is
one of the important ways by which the public health workforce can engage
with other sectors. HIA is not an established process in India although its
potential value has been identified (Caussy et al. 2003; Ahuja, 2007; Kumar et
al. 2011). The draft National Health Bill (MoHFW 2009) includes provisions
to make HIA mandatory for all new development projects but at the time of

writing this Bill had not passed into law. Environmental impact assessment (EIA) is, in contrast, well established. EIA is an important management tool for ensuring optimal use of natural resources for sustainable development (MoEF 2012). Indian EIA began with the assessment of river valley projects in 1978–1979 and currently encompasses sectors such as industry, power, and mining, all of which will have direct and indirect effects on population health. Therefore, the way that health is addressed in EIA provides an opportunity to explore the institutional and methodological implications of cross-sectoral work between the public health workforce and one sector of Indian planning, and it is a useful basis from which to identify actions to address current and emerging health challenges in India.

Case study: HIA and the consideration of health in EIAs in India

Methodology

Our research had three components and the results of each are reported below.

To establish a picture of HIA in India, we conducted an internet search for published examples of completed HIA reports and guidance. This focused on the term 'health impact assessment', ie it did not look for examples whereby health is included in other impact assessments (IAs).

To establish an understanding of the guidance that informs the ways in which EIAs are prepared we analysed the Ministry of Environment and Forests' (MoEF) guidance for EIA (2010a–j). We searched for occurrences of the word 'health' in the substantive text of the documents: the table of contents, acknowledgments, and bibliography were not included in this analysis nor were instances where 'health' did not refer to human health. We looked also at the *Draft Guidance Manual for Environmental Impact Assessment and Clearance of River Valley Projects* (MoEF 2009).

These results are considered in the light of a survey on the effectiveness of EIA in India and on the way in which EIA considers health. Three of the authors (Jha-Thakur, Labhasetwar, and Fischer) conducted this online survey between May 2011 and January 2012 (Jha-Thakur et al. unpublished). Key findings of this study are summarized below.

Results

HIA in India

Our search identified examples of HIA guidance, capacity building exercises, and reports.

Guidance: In 1992, the ADB established guidelines for HIA (Birley and Peralta 1992). HIA is required as part of the International Finance Corporation Performance Standards (IFC 2009). IAs from bank-funded projects are not in the public domain and do not feature in this review. The Central Public Health and Environmental Engineering Organization (CPHEEO) at the Ministry of Urban Development provided guidance on EIA and HIA with respect to municipal solid waste management (Shukla et al. 2000).

Capacity building: In 2003, the WHO published a training manual on inter-sectoral decision-making skills in support of HIA (Bos et al. 2003). This focused on water resource development projects and India was one of the five countries in which it was piloted. We are aware that training programmes for HIA in India have been conducted since 2003 (Martin Birley and Hilary Dreaves personal communication).

Reports: The National Institute of Malaria Research described four case studies (National Institute of Malaria Research 2009). Three were water resource development projects and involved epidemiological surveys of people living adjacent to existing projects. The fourth example described surveys and advice that informed the construction of a new line on the Konkan Railway. Cameron et al. (2011) described community-based HIAs in Kolkata, Patil (2011) reported the evaluation of the health and environmental effects of a mining operation, and Murthy et al. (2006) examined the effects of mining and focus on particular coal mines in Orissa. The Malaria Research Centre's (2009) water resource examples and Patil (2011) and Murthy et al. (2006) did not describe the potential effects of a proposed intervention but evaluated the existing effects of completed projects and so, strictly speaking, these analyses do not fulfil the criteria for HIAs.

EIA guidance and health

The Environment (Protection) Act (Government of India 1986) is concerned with minimizing environmental pollutants and hazardous substances, and with avoiding harm to human beings but human health is not explicitly mentioned. Health is, however, mentioned on 189 occasions in the substantive text of the ten MoEF guidance documents for EIA (2010a–j). These cover the following sectors: aerial ropeways, airports, asbestos-based industries, building construction and townships, coal washeries, highways, mineral beneficiation, mining, nuclear power plants, nuclear fuel processing plants, and nuclear waste management plants, and ports and harbours.

Table 13.1 shows the number of times that the word 'health' is mentioned in each of the guidance documents. It also shows how many times the word 'health' is mentioned in the sections that make up the guidance.

Table 13.1 Word count of 'health' in EIA guidance documents

MoEF Guidance document / Section in Guidance document	a	b	c	d	e	f	g	h	i	j	Total mentions by section
Introduction	-	-	1	-	-	-	-	1	-	-	2
Project description	-	-	-	-	-	-	-	-	-	-	1
Analysis of alternatives	-	1	-	-	-	-	-	-	1	-	1
Description of environment	2	2	1	6	2	3	4	2	4	3	29
Anticipated environmental impact and mitigation measures	5	5	-	6	1	3	1	4	-	4	29
Environmental monitoring program	-	-	1	-	-	-	-	4	-	-	5
Additional studies	-	2	18	-	-	-	1	1	6	1	29
Project benefits	-	1	-	-	1	-	1	1	-	1	5
Environmental CBA	-	-	-	-	-	-	-	-	-	-	0
Environmental management plan	1	-	-	-	-	-	-	7	-	-	8
Summary and conclusions	-	-	-	2	-	-	-	-	-	-	2
Disclosure of consultants engaged	-	-	-	-	-	-	-	-	-	-	0
Annexure	7	3	-	-	3	15	8	16	15	11	78
Total mentions by guidance document	15	14	21	14	7	21	15	36	26	20	189

(*Continued*)

Table 13.1 (*Continued*)

Key	
a	MoEF (2010a) *Environmental Impact Assessment Guidance Manual for Aerial Ropeways.*
b	MoEF (2010b) *Environmental Impact Assessment Guidance Manual for Airports.*
c	MoEF (2010c) *Environmental Impact Assessment Guidance Manual for Asbestos Based Industries.*
d	MoEF (2010d) *Environmental Impact Assessment Guidance Manual for Building, Construction, Townships and Area Development Projects.*
e	MoEF (2010e) *Environmental Impact Assessment Guidance Manual for Coal Washeries.*
f	MoEF (2010f) *Environmental Impact Assessment Guidance Manual for Highways.*
g	MoEF (2010g) *Environmental Impact Assessment Guidance Manual for Mineral Beneficiation.*
h	MoEF (2010h) *Environmental Impact Assessment Guidance Manual for Mining of Minerals.*
i	MoEF (2010i) *Environmental Impact Assessment Guidance Manual for Nuclear Power Plants, Nuclear Fuel Reprocessing Plants and Nuclear Waste Management Plants.*
j	MoEF (2010j) *Environmental Impact Assessment Guidance Manual for Ports and Harbors.*

The number of mentions ranges from 7 in the coal washeries guidance (MoEF 2010e) to 36 for the mining of minerals (MoEF 2010h). When health is mentioned it is usually in the context of ensuring that projects do no harm. Health is conceived as a property to be protected. The guidance documents focus on occupational health and safety: the examples that are provided in the text are mainly concerned with ensuring that people employed in the construction or operation of the projects are protected against injury. Project proponents are recommended to collect data on the health status of communities as part of the description of the environment so there is scope for expanding this view to include the wider community.

While the guidance is concerned with the wider socio-economic or socio-cultural effects of projects these are not consistently linked to potential health effects, beneficial or otherwise. There is some awareness of differential effect in that three of the guidance documents indicate that data on particular population groups should be gathered (see, for example, MoEF 2010f: 55; 2010g: 23; 2010i: 20). The guidance does not specify that health data should be collected for particular groups.

We turn now to the sections in which health is mentioned: Table 13.1 shows that these occur chiefly in the *Annexures*, the *Description of Environment* and the *Anticipated Environmental Impact and Mitigation Measures*. The *Annexures* revisit topics addressed earlier in the guidance documents and provide additional details so it is important that health is addressed in these sections. *Additional Studies* also has a high count for the word 'health' but this is somewhat skewed by the asbestos guidance.

EIAs are required to list the benefits that will accrue from project activities: five guidance manuals cite improvements in health as a possible benefit (MoEF 2010b,e,g, h,j). No indication is given as to how these benefits should be demonstrated.

If a benefit is to be claimed then it should also be followed up and monitored: human health is listed in the environmental management plan (EMP) of two documents (MoEF 2010a,d). The annexures describing the EMP for mining state that a plan for monitoring the health of workers and community in the vicinity should be drawn up and submitted along with a financial allocation (MoEF 2010g,h). The guidance for asbestos-based industries notes the value of, but stops short of requiring, health surveillance (MoEF 2010c: 2). The same guidance stipulates that additional studies should include the assessment of occupational health and it provides detail on monitoring the health of workers (MoEF 2010c: 54). The guidance for nuclear installations recommends epidemiological and health status surveys of the population living within a 30-km radius around the proposed site and for these to be repeated at 10-year intervals (MoEF 2010i: 34). The project proponent is advised to entrust this to the state health department or any reputed medical college and hospital. This is a rare example of a guidance manual directing the proponent to a health stakeholder. Health services for workers and for the wider community are mentioned as potential mitigation for project effects.

In closing we turn briefly to the *Draft Guidance Manual for Environmental Impact Assessment and Clearance of River Valley Projects* (MoEF 2009). This is structured differently to the guidance above. Health is still cast as a property to be protected but the guidance places health as a central concern of the EIA. It has references to health throughout its text and it directs the proponent to work with local health service units. This guidance also requires the preparation of a human health management plan, which must specify the costs of medical centres and surveys.

Results of the survey of health in EIAs

One hundred and seventy-nine EIA practitioners, researchers, and administrators participated in the online survey. We consider some of the results below.

Respondents were asked to choose one definition that reflects common understanding of health in Indian EIA practice. Thirty-six per cent described it as biophysical, focusing on environmental risks to human health. About one in four chose a comprehensive definition, describing it as a balanced state of well-being. Over half of the respondents felt that health should be addressed in EIA (Figure 13.1); only 20% thought this was not a good idea. Barriers included an inadequate definition of health, a rigid EIA process preventing a broader interpretation of health, and concern over political consequences.

Respondents were presented with a list of health issues covering biophysical aspects and social determinants of health. They were asked which were commonly addressed in EIA. There was a strong preference for socio-economic aspects, in particular employment, effects on the local economy, and education opportunities. Social infrastructure was also an issue, for example the availability of recreation areas and access to medical care, shops, and services. Non-biophysical aspects, for example mental health and behaviour, were rarely considered.

Respondents identified sources of health data as government agencies, research institutions (e.g. government hospitals, Indian Medical Association, Indian Council of Medical Research, and WHO), and medical journals.

The single most important barrier was the lack of adequate public awareness. It was also stated that competent authorities, project proponents, and

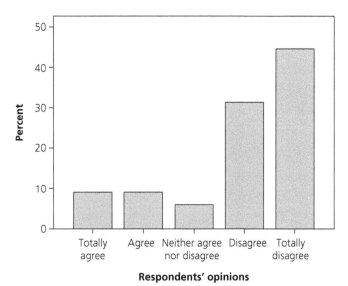

Fig. 13.1 Respondents' opinion on "Health should not be addressed in EIA".
Reproduced from Jha-Thakur, U., Fischer, T.B., Onyango, V., and Labhasetwar, P.,
Health within EIA in the UK and India: an international comparative study
(unpublished manuscript), University of Liverpool, copyright © 2012, with permission
of the author.

politicians withheld information in order to avoid public outcry. Structural
barriers included 'administrative loopholes' and 'competent authority inertia
to modify the regulations and guidelines'. Technical barriers included poorly
organized decision-making processes and inadequate research on causes and
effects. When asked how the barriers could be overcome, just over a quar-
ter of the respondents suggested that the EIA regulations and guidelines
should be improved and that there should be mandatory requirements for the
consideration of health in EIA (see Table 13.2). Other suggestions included
health-related training of EIA consultants, project proponents, and the general public. Political will and improved cooperation of EIA administrators was
vital. Finally, it was suggested that penalties for non-compliance could help
health to be more adequately considered.

Conclusions

With a growing population and a changing climate India faces existing and
new challenges to the state of her public's health. The approach to IA and
to HIA needs to reflect these changes. The results from this review accord
with international experience: human health is known to be affected by

Table 13.2 How can barriers to health inclusive EIA be overcome?

Suggestions	%
Improved and adequate regulation/guidance	26.9
Increased training/awareness/integrity among EIA consultants and project proponents	15.9
Raise public education, awareness, and levels of information about health issues within EIA	14.2
Increased political will and cooperation of EIA administrators	12.7
Increased public participation	11.1
Improved methodological framework and time to undertake extensive EIAs, including health issues	12.7
Integrate health experts within EIA practice	7.9
Transparency and access to quality data	6.3
Increased EIA research, showing cause and effect	4.6
Government to fund health mitigation costs instead of proponent	1.5
EIA to be administered by MoEF	1.5

Reproduced from Jha-Thakur, U., Fischer, T.B., Onyango, V., and Labhasetwar, P., Health within EIA in the UK and India: an international comparative study (unpublished manuscript), University of Liverpool, copyright © 2012, with permission of the author.

development (Ahuja 2007); environmental assessment, at strategic and at project level, provides opportunities for considering human health (Davies and Sadler 1997; Fischer et al. 2010; Harris-Roxas et al. 2012). These opportunities exist to different degrees within current and draft MoEF guidance documents. HIA, as a standalone process, also exists in India but is not firmly established.

A number of shortcomings were noted: our review of EIA guidance documents and our online survey highlighted that EIAs look at socio-economic and cultural effects of development but do not link these to health. Health is not explicitly defined. It tends to be addressed by teams with little or no expertise in human health. The focus tends to be restricted to occupational health or the provision of health services. These are clearly of great importance but this current focus must expand to address emerging challenges such as the growing burden posed by non-communicable diseases (NCDs) such as cardiovascular disease and cancer (WHO 2011; Prabhakaran et al. 2011). HIA, or a fuller incorporation of health into EIA, will bring new knowledge to the policy-maker and it can be expected to illuminate challenges such as mental ill health, NCDs, and health inequalities while also illuminating new solutions.

There is thus an opportunity to develop HIA to meet the challenges that India faces. Further avenues for exploration include ways in which to develop the requisite expertise among, and relationships between, the public health workforce and those involved in policy and development. IA in all forms is most effective when the policy-makers are aware of, and receptive to, the issues at hand. At minimum health stakeholders need to be involved in screening and scoping the assessments and in assuring the quality of completed reports. It will be important to identify ways in which HIA can be integrated into an institutional infrastructure that is currently struggling (Datta 2009; Sankhe et al. 2010), and ways to assure the transparency and the validity of IA reports when EIA practitioners, administrators, and researchers express concerns over the political consequences of their findings. In this chapter we focus on project-level considerations but similar observations apply to all levels of policy. These matters notwithstanding there are examples of HIAs and expertise across India, as well as opportunities to examine health within existing guidance. This is set against a background of demonstrable need and an increasing awareness of the importance of identifying the potential effects on the health of populations before the implementation of policies, plans, programmes, and projects.

Generic learning points

For public health practitioners and policy-makers

- EIA guidance contains many references to health. The opportunity exists to refine the approach currently taken and to include the social determinants of health and health inequalities.
- It would be opportune to develop capacity in anticipation of the draft National Health Bill (MoHFW 2009) passing into law.
- The public health workforce could build on the experience that exists, e.g. health input to water resource development. Developing health in EIA will help public health practitioners, policy-makers, and the public to work together to address important issues and create a stronger foundation for HIA in the future.
- A database of organizations with HIA expertise and a central repository of completed HIA (and related) reports will assist in developing capacity nationally and in ensuring that each state develops its own HIA resources.

For educators and researchers

Universities and institutions need inter-disciplinary curricula to overcome the current focus on science and engineering education in EIA in India and to strengthen the social science dimension (Gazzola 2009; Jha-Thakur 2011).

Inter-disciplinary research addressing existing and future challenges is essential in enhancing effective health consideration within planning. Core research teams should be developed which include experts from the fields of health, natural science, and the social sciences.

Bibliography

ADB (2012) *Asian Development Bank & India: Fact Sheet.* Manilla: Asian Development Bank. Available at <http://www.adb.org/publications/india-fact-sheet?ref=countries/india/publications>.

Ahuja, A. (2007) Health impact assessment in project and policy formulation. *Economic and Political Weekly* 42 (35): 3581–3587.

Birley, M. (2012) Personal correspondence, 3rd May 2012.

Birley, M.H. and Peralta, G.L. (1992) *Guidelines for the Health Impact Assessment of Development Projects.* ADB Environment Paper no 11. Manila: Asian Development Bank.

Bos, R., Birley, M., Furu, P., and Engel, C. (2003) *Health Opportunities in Development: A Course Manual on Developing Intersectoral Decision-making Skills in Support of Health Impact Assessment.* Geneva: WHO. Available at <http://www.who.int/water_sanitation_health/resources/hod/en/>.

Cameron, C., Ghosh, S., and Eaton, S.L. (2011) Facilitating communities in designing and using their own community health impact assessment tool. *Environmental Impact Assessment Review* 31 (4): 433–437.

Caussy, D., Kumar, P., and Than, S.U. (2003) Health impact assessment needs in south-east Asian countries. *Bulletin of the World Health Organization* 81 (6): 439–443.

Commission on the Social Determinants of Health (2008) *Closing the gap in a generation. Health equity through action on the social determinants of health.* Geneva: WHO. Available at <http://www.who.int/social_determinants/final_report/en/index.html>.

Datta, K.K. (2009) *Public Health Workforce in India: Career Pathways for Public Health Personnel.* Background paper for the National Consultation on Public Health Workforce in India. New Delhi: Ministry of Health & Family Welfare in collaboration with the WHO Country Office for India. Available at <http://bit.ly/PDH02R>.

Davies, K. and Sadler, B. (1997) *Environmental Assessment and Human Health: Perspectives, Approaches, and Future Directions.* Ottawa: Health Canada. Available at <http://www.bit.ly/JQozIB>.

Dreaves, H. (2012) Personal correspondence, 11th May 2012.

Fischer, T.B., Martuzzi, M., and Nowacki, J. (2010) The consideration of health in SEA. *Environmental Impact Assessment Review* 30 (3): 200–210.

Gazzola, P.and Jha-Thakur, U. (2009) Internationalisation and standardisation of European environmental assessment. Relevance to India. *Environmental Education Research* 15 (6): 25–641.

Government of India (1986) The Environment (Protection) Act. No. 29 of 1986. Available at <http://www.envfor.nic.in/legis/env/env1.html>.

Government of India (2011) Constitution of India. Updated up to (Ninety-Seventh Amendment) Act. Available at <http://www.indiacode.nic.in/coiweb/welcome.html>.

Harris-Roxas, B., Viliani, F., Bond, A., Cave, B., Divall, M., Furu, P., Harris, P., Soeberg, M., Wernham, A., and Winkler, M. (2012) Health impact assessment: the state of the art'. *Impact Assessment and Project Appraisal* 30 (1): 43–52.

IFC (2009) *Introduction to Health Impact Assessment.* Washington, DC: International Finance Corporation. Available at <http://www.bit.ly/wz8BkV>.

Jha-Thakur, U. (2011) Meeting success on the road less taken. *The Tribune.* Available at <http://www.tribuneindia.com/2011/20110928/jobs.htm#6>.

Jha-Thakur, U., Fischer, T. B., Onyango, V., and Labhasetwar, P. Health within EIA in the UK and India: an international comparative study (unpublished manuscript). University of Liverpool. 2012.

Kumar, A., Jain, R.B., Khanna, P., and Goel, M.K. (2011) Health impact assessment in India: need of the hour. *Internet Journal of Third World Medicine* 9 (2).

MoEF (2009) *Draft Guidance Manual for Environmental Impact Assessment and Clearance of River Valley Projects.* New Delhi: Government of India. Available at <http://www. bit.ly/KP4dCx>.

MoEF (2010a) *Environmental Impact Assessment Guidance Manual for Aerial Ropeways.* New Delhi: Ministry of Environment and Forests, Government of India. Available at <http://www.bit.ly/Ks7GjP>.

MoEF (2010b) *Environmental Impact Assessment Guidance Manual for Airports.* New Delhi: Government of India. Available at <http://www.bit.ly/Ks7GjP>.

MoEF (2010c) *Environmental Impact Assessment Guidance Manual for Asbestos Based Industries.* New Delhi: Government of India. Available at <http://www.bit.ly/ Ks7GjP>.

MoEF (2010d) *Environmental Impact Assessment Guidance Manual for Building, Construction, Townships and Area Development Projects.* New Delhi: Government of India. Available at <http://www.bit.ly/Ks7GjP>.

MoEF (2010e) *Environmental Impact Assessment Guidance Manual for Coal Washeries.* New Delhi: Government of India. Available at <http://www.bit.ly/Ks7GjP>.

MoEF (2010f) *Environmental Impact Assessment Guidance Manual for Highways.* New Delhi: Government of India. Available at <http://www.bit.ly/Ks7GjP>.

MoEF (2010g) *Environmental Impact Assessment Guidance Manual for Mineral Beneficiation.* New Delhi: Government of India. Available at <http://www.bit.ly/ Ks7GjP>.

MoEF (2010h) *Environmental Impact Assessment Guidance Manual for Mining of Minerals.* New Delhi: Government of India. Available at <http://www.bit.ly/Ks7GjP>.

MoEF (2010i) *Environmental Impact Assessment Guidance Manual for Nuclear Power Plants, Nuclear Fuel Reprocessing Plants and Nuclear Waste Management Plants.* New Delhi: Government of India. Available at <http://www.bit.ly/Ks7GjP>.

MoEF (2010j) *Environmental Impact Assessment Guidance Manual for Ports and Harbors.* New Delhi: Government of India. Available at <http://www.bit.ly/Ks7GjP>.

MoEF (2012) Environmental Impact Assessment (EIA) Division. New Delhi: Ministry of Environment and Forests, Government of India. Available at <http://www.moef.nic. in/modules/divisions/eia/>.

MoHFW (2009) *The National Health Bill*. Working draft—version January. New Delhi: Ministry of Health and Family Welfare, Government of India. Available at <http://www.bit.ly/MB1oRd>.

Murthy, A. and Patra, H.S. (2006) *Ecological, Socio-economic & Health Impact Assessment due to Coal Mining—A Case Study of Talabira Coal Mines in Orissa*. Vasundhara, Bhubaneshwar: Conservation & Livelihood Team. Available at <http://www.bit.ly/IwIqun>.

National Institute of Malaria Research (2009) Health impact assessment (HIA) of development projects with reference to mosquito-borne diseases, in Dash, A.P. (ed.), *A Profile of the National Institute of Malaria Research*, 2nd edition. New Delhi: Indian Council of Medical Research. Available at <http://www.bit.ly/JNE1T1>.

Patil, R.R. (2011) Environmental health impact assessment of National Aluminum Company, Orissa. *Indian Journal of Occupational & Environmental Medicine* 15 (2): 73–75.

Prabhakaran, D., Ajay, V.S., Mohan, V., Thankappan, K.R., Siegel, K., Venkat Narayan, K.M., and Reddy, K.S. (2011) Chronic diseases in India, in Stuckler, D. and Siegel, K. (eds), *Sick Societies: Responding to the Global Challenge of Chronic Disease*. Oxford: Oxford University Press.

Quigley, R., den Broeder, L., Furu, P., Bond, A., Cave, B., and Bos, R. (2006) *Health Impact Assessment*. International Association for Impact Assessment, International best practice principles. Special publication series No. 5. Available at <http://www.iaia.org/publicdocuments/special-publications/SP5.pdf>.

Sankhe, S., Vittal, I., Dobbs, R., Mohan, A., Gulati, A., Ablett, J., Gupta, S., Kim, A., Paul, S., Sanghvi, A., Sethy, G. (eds) (2010) *India's urban awakening: building inclusive cities, sustaining economic growth*. Seoul, London, Mumbai: McKinsey Global Institute. Available at <http://www.bit.ly/LCZMWG>.

Shukla, S.R., Akolkar, A.B., Bhide, A.D., Dhussa, A.K., Varshney, A.K., Acharya, D.B., Datta, M.M., Dutta, M., Mazumdar, N.B., Asnani, P.U., Ramanathan, R., Ramaprasad, V.B., Uppal, B.B., and Dhinadhayalan, M (eds) (2000) *Manual on municipal solid waste management*. New Delhi: Central Public Health and Environmental Engineering Organisation, Ministry of Urban Development. Available at <http://www.indiawater-portal.org/taxonomy/term/6212>.

WHO (2011) Global status report on noncommunicable diseases: 2010. Geneva, Switzerland. Available at <http://whqlibdoc.who.int/publications/2011/9789240686458_Eng.pdf>.

WHO and United Nations Human Settlements Programme (2010) *Hidden Cities: Unmasking and Overcoming Health Inequities in Urban Settings*. Kobe: WHO Centre for Health Development and Geneva: United Nations Human Settlements Programme (UN-HABITAT). Available at <http://www.hiddencities.org/downloads/WHO_UN-HABITAT_Hidden_Cities_Web.pdf>.

Chapter 14

Realities and opportunities for health impact assessment in Africa

Francesca Viliani and Edith Essie Clarke

This chapter begins by analysing the historical evolution of health impact assessment (HIA) in Africa. It then briefly presents what is happening nowadays, and finally provides a set of learning points that might assist in strengthening the practice in the continent.

HIA in Africa has mainly been carried out in relation to infrastructure projects, and even for these projects it has not been done in a systematic and integrated way. Although authorities were aware that project development and man-made environmental change generates health consequences, this knowledge has not been easily transformed into project safeguards. Furthermore, the main focus historically has been on communicable diseases, while other health impacts and equity considerations have not been fully addressed. Finally, inter-sectoral policy dialogue and decision-making have only recently become a priority for national governments. This will influence HIA practice in the continent. In order to achieve the successful use of HIA at project and policy level, lessons from the past need to be learned and transformed into new settings for the use of HIA in the future.

Historical application and the use of HIA in Africa

The history of HIA in Africa goes back several decades (Macdonald 1955) and has been profoundly shaped by some of the main features of the continent, such as the need for development and infrastructure projects, the high burden of communicable diseases, which is closely linked to the richness and fragility of African ecosystems, its high mineral and natural resource development potential, and the presence of international actors and donors.

Development and infrastructure projects (agriculture development, hydropower, and mining)

HIA in Africa began by focusing on water use associated with agricultural development projects and dams for the generation of hydropower constructed across the continent. For a long time, national governments and agricultural policies were centred on the positive effects of these projects, such as improved nutritional security and increased trade and export. However, already in the 1950s it was quite clear that the irrigation systems and large dams were also bringing with them negative health consequences, for example an increase of vector-borne diseases, malnutrition, psycho-social disorders, and so on. Large hydropower projects are among the most environmentally and socially complex types of projects (Scudder 2005: 52) and therefore have attracted considerable public interest and have substantially advanced the practice and use of impact assessment (IA).

The mix of positive and negative impacts associated with development projects and policies are the cornerstone of HIA history in Africa. In fact, a guideline to support the design of development programmes and projects so as to have a favourable impact on health was developed by the end of the 1970s (Barbiero 1979). Economic sectors and development policies (Cooper Weil et al. 1990) were initially perceived as exclusively positive forces for development and change, while their associated negative social, environmental, and health consequences were appraised and considered only at a later stage, often after the project had been granted permission or the policy had been implemented. This decision-making approach inadvertently transfers the costs of the negative impacts to the local community and to the health system, and quite often in an unequal way, as disadvantaged groups are disproportionately affected (Quigley et al. 2006).

It is widely accepted that changes to the environment and social situation always generate a change in health status and 'ironically, economic activity under the banner of development often created ill health' (Hunter et al. 1982: 1135). A further complication in the continent emerged through the rapid and uncontrolled/unplanned urbanization process, where the poor environmental situation coupled with social contexts of disadvantage (Stephens 1995) favoured a further increase of inequality. In this context, the need for a transparent and open HIA process is essential to ensure that the positive, as well as the negative, health consequences associated with a sector or a policy are jointly addressed in a timely manner.

High burden of communicable diseases

Another characteristic of HIA practice in the African continent is the focus on communicable diseases. The importance of the ecosystem in regulating and influencing the burden of infectious diseases, as well as providing a wealth of services to human populations, is widely accepted (Corvalan et al. 2005). The role of the ecosystem services as a complex web of determinants of health and human wellbeing in different African contexts is even more relevant than in other geographical regions as the ecosystem is still a major provider of services for local communities. In Africa, around 31% of the disease burden is attributable to environmental factors. This is the highest percentage in the world (Prüss-Ustün and Corvalan 2006). Furthermore, Africa, together with South-East Asia, bears 54% of the total global burden of disease, although they account for only about 40% of the world's population (WHO 2008).

The first issues identified and researched as key priorities were vector-borne diseases (Stanley and Alpers 1975), with a focus on schistosomiasis (Jobin et al. 1976) and malaria (Keiser et al. 2005). For these reasons, guidelines (Birley 1991; Tiffen 1991) on how to include health safeguards in irrigation and other water resource development projects were developed by the Joint WHO/FAO/UNEP/UNCHS Panel of Experts on Environmental Management (PEEM) for vector control. While the panel was not focusing specifically on Africa, much of the research and evidence used as input to the guidelines came from the African continent.

By the 1990s, it was quite clear that health impacts and opportunities associated with development projects were multiple and were both direct and indirect; most importantly they could be predicted and therefore addressed during the project design phase (Konradsen et al. 1997). The driving forces leading to health impacts were broadly categorized as environmental, ecological, demographic, and socioeconomic changes (WHO 1997). For example, the health consequences of agricultural projects were not limited to vector-borne diseases. Among other factors considered were the negative effects due to the improper use of pesticides (Bull 1982), the negative psychosocial effects due to displacement and relocation because of dam construction (Cernea and McDowell 2000), and nutritional status. At the same time, the health consequences of other development projects were slowly being understood. For example, the increase in schistosomiasis prevalence in a mining area of the Democratic Republic of Congo was associated with ecological changes created by mine construction and operation (Polderman 1986).

Nevertheless, it was only with the emergence and spread of HIV/AIDS in the continent and the recognition of its impact on business (Baggaley et al. 1995) that the practice to more explicitly consider health issues in the context of large-scale development projects was achieved. Unfortunately, this left the impression that health impacts were mainly associated with HIV/AIDS and a few vector-borne diseases. Thus these have often been the main—or only—health issues addressed in integrated impact assessment (IIA) in the continent. In other words, this limited the understanding of the need to consider how projects impact wider health determinants and health outcomes.

Presence and influence of international actors and donors

The practice of including health considerations within environmental impact assessment (EIA) in the continent is not casual and has been supported by national governments, as well as by development agencies and academic institutions. Indeed, almost simultaneously to the Gothenburg meeting (WHO-ECHP 1999) another meeting took place in Arusha, Tanzania (WHO 2001) to explore the most effective ways of strengthening the capacity of African countries in HIA, where it was decided that HIA practice would be developed in the context of the already existing frameworks of environmental regulations.

EIA, in contrast to HIA, is a legal requirement for projects in the whole continent, so environmental protection agencies or departments exist in each African country and are responsible for EIA. The basic steps of EIA and HIA are similar, but EIA tends to focus to a greater extent on the biophysical domain. This is mainly because there is a lack of internal capacity within environmental bodies for considering health in a comprehensive way. Therefore the EIA processes have resulted in limited coverage of health, largely focusing only on environmental determinants such as air, water, and so on. At the same time, the health sector has thus far not been able to utilize these planning and assessment opportunities as important entry points for influencing determinants of health as well as primary prevention of disease. Today, the largest portion of the health development funds and budget allocations either support the curative domain of the health system or support vertical control programmes. These funds cannot readily be used to build capacity in health in all policy (HiAP) or inter-sectoral collaboration within and beyond the Ministry of Health.

The WHO and other organizations have made a significant attempt to address this lack of capacity and have developed and carried out several training courses in Africa over the last two decades, starting with a focus on health opportunities in water resources development. These experiences led to the development of a manual called *Developing Intersectoral Decision-Making Skills in Support of Health Impact Assessment* (Bos et al. 2003). This manual was based on the conviction that IA procedures are crucial in the planning of development projects, especially if planners and governments are interested in sustainability and human wellbeing. The use of the word 'opportunities' instead of 'impacts' was adopted in order to focus on the broad spectrum of possibilities associated with development projects and policies, rather than exclusively on the negative consequences. This understanding and support for IA in general finally led to the inclusion of health considerations within EIA of projects instead of developing specific requirements and tools for HIA, although this inclusion has never been systematically and consistently achieved.

High mineral and natural resource development potential

The first project for which there exists extensive documentation about the inclusion of health considerations in EIA is the Chad-Cameroon Petroleum Development and Pipeline project, for which construction started in 2000. This project was the biggest energy project with both private and public financial support developed in the African continent at that time. Moreover, the system devised for the IA process and its follow-up were quite innovative. Unfortunately, the results of the EIA process and especially the follow-up procedure were unsatisfactory (Jobin 2003), highlighting the challenges associated with the IA of complex projects. Some of the key problems identified in the project included the difficulties in proposing alternatives to the proposed project activities accepted by all parties, the challenge of conducting iterative IA when project design changes over time, the lack of full accountability for the implementation of mitigation measures when multiple stakeholders are responsible for different components, and finally poor monitoring and evaluation of recommendations when no budget for these monitoring activities has been allocated and no penalties or incentives exist to execute the follow-up programme (Viliani 2005).

The presence of large multi-national corporations investing heavily in mining and oil and gas projects in the continent has also made an important contribution to the development of HIA practice. Private companies have increasingly commissioned HIA as either standalone assessment or as a component of the integrated assessment of their projects even where this was not a national requirement. The reasons usually correspond to one or more of the following points:

- company policies on corporate social responsibilities and/or sustainable development
- industrial regulation and standards on community health
- obtaining and maintaining the social license to operate in given communities
- risk characterization and management to reduce possible litigation and reputational problems

- the impact of health of the community reflects on the health of the work-force, and the importance of reducing absenteeism and medical costs
- international financing.

Access to financial support from both national governments and private companies is in fact one of the key drivers of HIA development in the continent. The World Bank Group provides, amongst other things, financial support to national governments, as well as to private companies interested in infrastructure and investment projects. The World Bank has been involved for decades in many of the major African hydro-development projects, which means that they have brought in a culture of EIA and a focus on social IA. The group has for a long time attempted to incorporate environmental health into project design through several publications (Birley et al. 1997; Listorti and Doumani 2001) and through the constant update of their environmental and social safeguard policies. The African Development Bank includes health considerations as an interwoven theme in the integrated environmental and social impact assessment (IESIA) guidelines and highlights the importance of understanding health as a 'multidimensional concept' that is not limited to the absence of disease and infirmity but a status strongly affected by changes in the determinants of health (AfDB 2003).

The latest example is the International Finance Corporation (IFC) Performance Standards (PS), which define clients' roles and responsibilities for managing their projects (IFC 2012). IFC is the branch of the World Bank Group providing financial assistance to the private sector, while other members of the group work closely with national governments. The IFC PS number 4 deals specifically with community health, safety, and security. The IFC PS has been developed to assess the potential consequences of specific and individual projects that are mainly financed by private investors. Therefore the IFC PS adopts a risk management approach to IA, as their main users are private companies and not national governments.

Current HIA developments in Africa

Many of the challenges encountered in the practice of HIA in the African continent in the past are still present today. These include the need for a more systematic use of HIA at policy or project design stage, the challenges of inter-sectoral collaboration, the lack of resources to carry out and evaluate HIA or including health considerations in EIA, and the scarcity of reliable health baseline information to carry out pre- and post-intervention evaluations (Appiah-Opoku 2001; WHO-UNEP 2008a)(Appiah-Opoku 2001; WHO 2001; WHO 2008).

The situation is, however, changing and in August 2008 in Libreville (Gabon) the first Inter-ministerial Conference on Health and Environment in Africa convened. The aim of this conference was to secure political commitment among African governments, which was needed to reduce environmental threats to health in order to realize sustainable development. The main output of the conference was the Libreville Declaration, which includes HIA as one of the 10 priorities. Point number 9 of the declaration specifically calls on national governments and international organizations to institute 'the practice of systematic assessment of health and environment risks, in particular through the development of procedures to assess impacts on health' (WHO-UNEP 2008b). This call has been reconfirmed at the Second Inter-ministerial Conference, which took place in Luanda (Angola) in November 2011, at which a side event about HIA was jointly organized by WHO, the Ghana Health Service, and the Ghana Environmental Protection Agency.

As part of the Libreville Process, countries conducted situation analysis and needs assessment on the Libreville Declaration on health and environmental inter-linkages. One of the key findings was that most countries have in place environmental legislation and permit procedures requiring the systematic assessment of the environmental and social impacts of projects. However, provisions for the systematic assessment of health impacts within this existing framework are urgently needed. Another challenge is the lack of inter-sectoral integrated efforts in planning and research. This is often due to weak arrangements and requirements for cooperation as well as a long established independent and non-collaborative attitude and practice of national institutions and departments, reinforced by similarly siloed funding mechanisms. Therefore, there is a need for dedicated financial resources for inter-sectoral decision-making and for developing detailed and specific frameworks for undertaking strategic HIA or inclusion of health in SEA at the policy and planning level.

Agriculture, general infrastructure, mining, and oil and gas continue to be major investment priorities in most of the African continent. There will be more complicated and large-scale development projects to come. An increasing number of these will be funded by donors and investors that do not have the same environmental, social protection, and precautionary culture.

Conclusion

The practice of HIA in Africa is not new and goes back several decades, as shown in Figure 14.1.

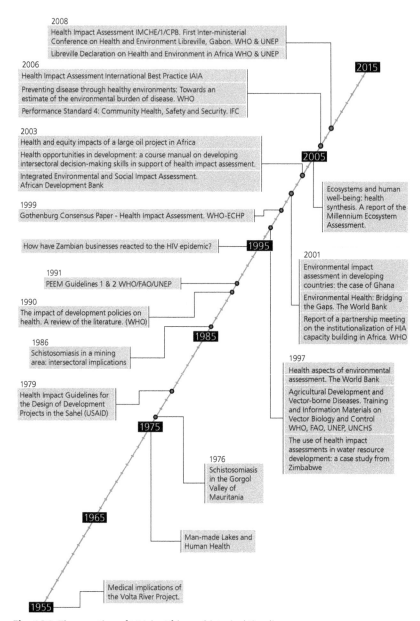

Fig. 14.1 The practice of HIA in Africa: a historical timeline.

This practice has been widely supported, and therefore influenced, by the international development community. As such, it has focused mainly on the inclusion of health considerations within EIA and has concentrated on specific development projects. However, the health systems in Africa have not been able to use the EIA process in order to fully and systematically address the health consequences of the projects under scrutiny and they have struggled to work in closer collaboration with the environmental agencies. The negative health impacts associated with the projects under assessment have therefore not been adequately identified, managed, and monitored.

This situation is now changing. Health and environmental inter-linkages are an important item on the agenda of national governments across the African continent. Efforts are being made to include health considerations more broadly and systematically in the IA process. Furthermore, this approach is not limited to projects; through SEA the health consequences of the main economic sectors in the continent are also assessed. The application of HIA at a strategic level provides potential opportunities for more in-depth assessment of health impacts at the sector level through a process of strategic health impact assessment (sHIA), employing steps similar to those of the SEA. A number of African countries have expressed an interest in applying the principles of sHIA in the extractive industry sector based on guidelines recently developed by WHO. Ghana is leading the way as it has already set the process in motion.

To ensure that new investments bring positive health outcomes and wellbeing to the countries where investments are being made, the lessons learned from the past should inform the future applications of HIA.

Generic learning points

For public health practitioners and policy makers

◆ National ministries of health must actively drive, with the environmental agencies, the IA process and simultaneously build the capacity and resources necessary to ensure adequate implementation and follow up. However, to do this they have to be mandated and capacitated to play this role.

◆ National governments should develop their own frameworks and requirements for HIA and not just rely on IFC PS and industry-specific standards on community health protection.

◆ The development community can contribute to this process by further supporting capacity development for HIA and by providing support for establishing the enabling conditions needed for institutionalizing HIA.

- ◆ The HIA process should be subject to the same information disclosure requirements as other IA and EIA processes. A transparent and open HIA process is essential to assure that the positive, as well as the negative, health consequences associated with a sector or a policy are jointly and timely addressed.

- ◆ Follow-up and monitoring of the results of HIA, both on specific projects and more broadly (i.e. in terms of uptake and national practice), is critical to ensuring the quality of HIAs carried out as well as ensuring that the investments and application of HIA is generating the intended or desired result.

For educators and researchers

- ◆ More research on how health can be better included in EIA and SEA in the African context is needed.

- ◆ Equity considerations should be included and considered throughout the process to ensure that disadvantaged groups are not disproportionately affected. To achieve this we need to gain a better visibility and understanding of equity in the African context.

- ◆ Capacity-building activities and strategies cannot just be replicated but need to be contextualized and adapted.

References

AfDB (2003) *Integrated Environmental and Social Impact Assessment*. African Development Bank.

Appiah-Opoku, S. (2001) Environmental impact assessment in developing countries: the case of Ghana. *Environmental Impact Assessment Review* 21(1): 59–71.

Baggaley, R., Godfrey-Faussett, P., Msiska, R., Chilangwa, D., Chitu, E., Porter, J. and Kelly, M. (1995) How have Zambian businesses reacted to the HIV epidemic? *Occupational and Environmental Medicine* 52: 565–569.

Barbiero, V. (1979) *Health Impact Guidelines for the Design of Development Projects in the Sahel: Volume 1: Sector-specific Reviews and Methodology*. Washington, DC: Family Health Care Inc & United States Agency for International Development (USAID).

Birley, M. (1991) *Guidelines for Forecasting the Vector-borne Disease Implications of Water Resources Development*. WHO/CWS/91.3. PEEM Guidelines. Geneva: WHO.

Birley, M., Gomes, M. and Davy, A. (1997) *Health aspects of environmental assessment*. Environmental Assessment Sourcebook Update 18. Washington, DC: Environmental Division, The World Bank.

Bos, R., Birley, M., Furu, P. and Engel, C. (2003) *Health opportunities in development: a course manual on developing intersectoral decision-making skills in support of health impact assessment*. Geneva: WHO, Liverpool School of Tropical Medicine, Danish Bilhrarziasis Laboratory, Institute of Education University of London.

Bull, D. (1982) *A growing problem, pesticides and the world poor.* Oxford: Oxfam.

Cernea, M. M. and Mcdowell, C. (2000) *Risks and Reconstruction: experiences of resettlers and refugees.* Washington DC: The World Bank.

Cooper Weil, D., Alicbusan, A.P., Wilson, J., Reich, M. and Bradley, D. (1990) *The impact of development policies on health. A review of the literature.* Geneva: WHO.

Corvalan, C., Hales, S. and McMichael, A. (2005) *Ecosystems and human well-being: health synthesis.* A report of the Millennium Ecosystem Assessment. Geneva: WHO.

Hunter, J. M., Rey, L. and Scott, D. (1982) Man-made lakes and man-made diseases. Towards a policy resolution. *Social Science and Medicine* 16: 1127–1145.

IFC (2012) *Performance Standard 4: Community Health, Safety and Security.* Washington, DC: International Finance Corporation.

Jobin, W. (2003) Health and equity impacts of a large oil project in Africa. *Bulletin of the World Health Organization* 81: 420–426.

Jobin, W. R., Negron-Aponte, H. and Michelson, E.H. (1976) Schistosomiasis in the Gorgol Valley of Mauritania. *American Journal of Tropical Medicine and Hygiene* 25: 587–594.

Keiser, J., De Castro, M.C., Maltese, M.F., Bos, R., Tanner, M., Singer, B.H. and Utzinger, J. (2005) Effect of irrigation and large dams on the burden of malaria on a global and regional scale. *American Journal of Tropical Medicine and Hygiene* 72: 392–406.

Konradsen, F., Chimbari, M., Furu, P., Birley, M.H. and Christensen, N.O. (1997) The use of health impact assessments in water resource development: a case study from Zimbabwe. *Impact Assessment* 15: 55–72.

Listorti, J.A. and Doumani, F.M. (2001) Environmental Health: Bridging the Gaps. Washington, DC: The World Bank.

Macdonald, G. (1955) Medical implications of the Volta River Project. *Transactions of the Royal Society of Tropical Medicine and Hygiene* 49: 13–27.

Polderman, A.M. (1986) Schistosomiasis in a mining area: intersectoral implications. *Tropical Medicine and Parasitology* 37: 195–199.

Prüss-Ustün, A and Corvalan, C. (2006) Preventing disease through healthy environments: Towards an estimate of the environmental burden of disease Geneva: WHO.

Quigley, R. Den Broeder, L. Furu, P., Bond, A. Cave, B. and Bos, R. (2006) *Health Impact Assessment International Best Practice Principles.* Special Publication Series No. 5. Fargo: USA International Association for Impact Assessment.

Scudder, T. (2005) *The Future of Large Dams: Dealing with Social, Environmental, Institutional and Political Costs.* London: Earthscan.

Stanley, N.F. and Alpers, M.P. (eds) (1975) *Man-made Lakes and Human Health* London, New York, San Francisco: Academic Press Inc.

Stephens, C. (1995) The urban environment, poverty and health in developing countries. *Health Policy Plan* 10: 109–121.

Tiffen, M. (1991) *Guidelines for the Incorporation of Health Safeguards into Irrigation Projects through Intersectoral Cooperation with special reference to the vector-borne diseases.* WHO/CWS/91.2 PEEM Guidelines. Geneva: WHO.

Viliani, F. (2005) *Health impact assessment of extractive industries in developing countries: how to address STI and HIV/AIDS risk factors.* London: London School of Hygiene and Tropical Medicine.

WHO (1997) *Agricultural Development and Vector-borne Diseases. Training and Information Materials on Vector Biology and Control.* Slide Set Series. Geneva: WHO, FAO, UNEP, UNCHS.

WHO (2001) *Report of a partnership meeting on the institutionalization of HIA capacity building in Africa.* WHO/SDE/WSH/01.07. Geneva: WHO.

WHO (2008) *The global burden of disease: 2004 update.* Geneva: WHO.

WHO-ECHP (1999) *Gothenburg Consensus Paper—Health Impact Assessment. Main concepts and suggested approach.* Copenhagen: WHO.

WHO-UNEP (2008a) *Health Impact Assessment IMCHE/1/CP8. First Inter-ministerial Conference on Health and Environment Libreville, Gabon.* WHO/UNEP.

WHO-UNEP (2008b) *Libreville Declaration on Health and Environment in Africa.* Available at <http://www.afro.who.int/en/clusters-a-programmes/hpr/protection-of-the-human-environment.html>. Brazzaville: WHO Regional Office for Africa.

Chapter 15

Implementing and institutionalizing health impact assessment in Spain: challenges and opportunities

Piedad Martín-Olmedo

Introduction

The use of health impact assessment (HIA) has grown steadily as governments have increasingly placed public health issues high on their agendas. HIA provides a structured framework that helps policy-makers estimate the potential consequences that health and non-health sector policies can have on overall community health, ultimately maximizing health gains and contributing, whenever possible, to reducing health inequalities.

The affinity of HIA with the European health in all policies (HiAP) strategy (Ståhl et al. 2006) strengthens current opportunities for the implementation of this tool in Spain, particularly in the context of current debate on the future of public health and the need to ensure that it acquires a higher priority on political-institutional agendas.

This chapter analyses Spanish efforts to broaden HIA's implementation and institutionalization while summarizing experiences conducted by regional and local administrations as well as research groups. Institutionalization is defined as the systematic integration of HIA into the decision-making process (Wismar et al. 2007). This chapter will describe how HIA is being incorporated into recent Spanish national and regional public health laws as a means to encourage more successful inter-sectoral health actions. It will also address questions and opinions raised by key informants regarding possible challenges and hurdles associated with this process.

Data on HIA institutionalization in Spain was gathered through a literature review of case studies and legislative documents referring to HIA or HiAP, as well as a semi-structured questionnaire sent by email to 21 key informants employed by research institutions or central and regional public health administration. The search strategy involved interrogation in Google and PubMed using the free text terms ['health impact assessment' AND 'Spain'] for case studies, and ['law' AND 'public health' or 'health'] by each of the regions within Spain for legal documents. E-mail survey participants were deliberately chosen based on their previous experience in HIA, and from the attendance list of an annual international conference held in Granada (13–14 April 2011), the largest gathering of HIA practitioners in Spain. The question-naire sought information on published and unpublished HIA experiences, as well as perceived benefits and hurdles linked to HIA's potential mandatory institutionalization in Spain.

Background

HIA experience in Spain

Results show that most of the Spanish experience on HIA was conducted on an ad hoc basis, financed mainly through research funding. Fifteen different practical initiatives (Table 15.1) were identified, some containing several case studies (i.e. Apheis or Aphekom projects). The most prominent sectors were air quality and urban planning. Only two initiatives (González-Enríquez et al. 2002; Boldo et al. 2011) were conducted at the national level, the rest were performed in local settings. In a larger sample of case studies run worldwide, Davenport et al. (2006) reported similar findings and argued that national policies or programmes were less likely to be assessed due to their complexity and greater uncertainty regarding potential impacts. In the HIA procedure's 'appraisal stage' (Kemm 2007), a technical rational methodology was usu-ally applied in the Spanish initiatives linked to environmental health deter-minants (Table 15.1), with emphasis on methods for quantifying the health benefits obtained when certain risk factors were reduced (i.e. ambient levels of fine particulates). HIA case studies conducted in other sectors have focused on participatory approaches and a broader view of health by applying qualita-tive assessment methodologies. Table 15.1 also provides an overview of the few activities undertaken in Spain to promote capacity building and HIA intelligence.

Current initiatives for HIA institutionalization in Spain

The conceptual framework used by Wismar et al. (2007) proposed four major categories to analyse the diverse forms for attaining HIA implementation and institutionalization across Europe: stewardship, financing, resource genera-tion, and technical leadership for delivering.

Table 15.1 HIA initiatives (case studies/guidelines/training) identified in Spain

Topic	HIA case studies (most recent reference)[4]	Region
Urban planning	Regeneration plan of Uretamendi-Betolaza[3,4] (Bacigalupe et al. 2010)	BC
	Palma beach regeneration project[1] (ongoing) <http://www.lasalutentot.org/>	BI
	Regeneration project in Alcalá de Guadaíra[3] (Venegas et al. 2011)	A
	Tunnelling of the railroad in Vitoria-Gasteiz[2,4] (Gómez and Estibalez 2011)	BC
Housing improvement	Rehabilitation measures in a Barcelona neighborhood[3,4] (Morteruel and Díez 2011)	C
Atmospheric air pollution	Ambient air and health in Barcelona's metropolitan area[1] (Kunzli and Pérez 2007)	C
	Apheis project[3,4] (<http://www.apheis.org>)	A, BC, C, M, V
	APHEKOM project[3,4] (<http://www.aphekom.org>; Martín-Olmedo et al. 2011)	A, BC, C, V
	SERCA project[3] (ongoing) (Boldo et al. 2011)	National
	HEREPLUS project[1] (<http://www.hereplusproject.eu/>)	M
Transport	Assessment of Granada City's metro line[3] (González et al. 2007)	A
	Biking in Barcelona[3] (Rojas-Rueda et al. 2011)	C
Smoking policy	Implementing a smoking cessation intervention in Spain[2] (González-Enríquez et al. 2002)	National
	A private sector initiative: a smoke-free workplace policy[2,4] (Barroso 2007)	C
Health inequalities	URBACT—Building healthy communities[1] (ongoing) (<http://www.urbact.eu/>)	M
Other initiatives		
Guidelines	First guidelines for HIA in Spanish[3] (Rueda 2005)	BC
Training	Introductory courses for public health officers[1] (five editions)	A, BC, BI
Tools	▪ Screening tools for regional policies in the BC[3] (Aldasoro 2009) ▪ Screening tool for regional policies in A[1] (pending publication) ▪ Online tool for conducting HIA[1] (<http://www.lasalutentot.org/>)	BC A BI

[1]Derived from email survey only; [2]derived from case study review only; [3]derived from more than one source; [4]several published documents exist related to this initiative, but only most recent were recorded.

A: Andalusia; BC: Basque Country; BI: Balearic Islands; C: Catalonia; M: Community of Madrid; V: Community of Valencia

Policy formulation is one of the tasks comprising the category 'stewardship' (Wismar et al. 2007). According to some authors, the existence of a legislative framework for HIA would provide permanent rules and legitimacy for HIA within the policy process (Banken 2001; Metcalfe and Higgins 2009; Kearns and Pursell 2011).

Articles 148.1.21 and 149.1.16 of the Spanish Constitution (1978) provide that responsibilities on health issues be shared between the State and the country's autonomous regions. The former recognizes the authority of local regions on questions related to 'health and hygiene' while the latter reserves exclusive powers to the State for issues affecting 'the health system's legal basis and overall coordination', among others. The premise of article 149.1.16 is that the State must harmonize key elements to ensure the highest protection of all Spanish citizens' constitutional right to health (article 43). Through this division of powers, a minimal framework is established under national law to facilitate coordination and cooperation on public health issues among the different Administrations; those actions can later be regulated more extensively in accordance with statutes applicable in each specific region.

A total of 11 regulatory documents that explicitly or implicitly encourage institutionalization of HIA in Spain were identified (Table 15.2). Most of these regulations have been approved very recently. Generally speaking, all of them recognize the need to improve the population's health through interventions and policies not exclusively limited to the health sector. In this sense, the principle of equality and HiAP, as well as a review of the best available scientific evidence prior to the actual decision-making process, is addressed directly. Similarly, all documents strongly emphasize cross-sectional, participative, and inter-sectoral strategies to ensure the highest possible degree of efficacy in meeting public health goals.

Eight of the 11 documents included HIA as an instrument for materializing HiAP strategy, but only three of them (National, Andalusia, and Basque Country) introduce a mandatory requirement to conduct prospective evaluations of sectoral public policies. A more open-ended formula, with a voluntary application of HIA, is chosen by Catalonia and the Balearic Islands in their respective public health laws. As the literature reflects, mandatory inclusion of HIA remains a controversial issue. Some authors believe that social and economic relevance of non-health-related policies make it essential for HIA practice to be mandatory (Mannheimer et al. 2007; Oxman et al. 2010; Smith et al. 2010). Kemm (2007) also suggested that were HIA to become legally binding then faulty HIA could be subject to prosecution, which in turn would encourage more robust HIA practices. Critics, however, believe that without political and logistical consensus, legislative mandates would simply convert HIA into

Table 15.2 Policy regulations that provide a framework for HIA institutionalization in Spain

Region	Reference document	Type of HIA endorsement*	Scope for HIA application
National	Law 33/2011, General Public Health Act[1] (BOE 240, 5 October 2011)	A-M	Public interventions**
Andalusia	Regional Public Health Act[1] (BOJA 255, 31 December 2011)	A-M	Public interventions**; urban planning projects; public or private interventions linked to environmental impact assessment regulation; others***
Aragon	Regional Public Health Bill (January 2011)	A-M	Undefined
Balearic Islands	Law 16/2010 of Public Health[1] (BOE 30, 4 February 2011)	A-NM	Undefined
Basque Country	Regional Public Health draft bill[2]	A-M	Public interventions**
Castilla-La Mancha	Regional Public Health draft bill[2]	A-NM	Undefined
Castilla-Leon	Law 10/2010 of Public Health and Food Safety[1] (BOE 283, 23 November 2010)	NA-HiAP	—
Catalonia	Law 18/2009 of Public Health[1] (BOE 276, 16 November 2010)	A-NM	Undefined
Extremadura	Law 7/ 2011 of Public Health[1] (BOE 88, 13 April 2011)	NA-HiAP	—
Navarra	Law 17/2010 of Health matters[1] (BOE 315, 28 December 2010)	NA-HiAP	—
Valencia	Health Promotion draft bill[2]	A-NM	Undefined

[1]Documents already approved and officially published; [2]documents unavailable, information provided by email survey.

A-NM: HIA is specifically addressed but its application would not be mandatory; A-M: HIA is specifically addressed and its application is compulsory under a defined scope; NA-HiAP: HIA is not specifically addressed but the document refers to principles of Health in All Policies and health inequalities.

Public interventions refer to policies, projects or programs for which public administrations require the submission of HIA (health and non-health policies). Others refer to specific activities that could affect public health and would be defined and addressed by specific regulations in the future.

BOE refers to the Spanish Official legislative bulletin; BOJA refers to the Andalusian Official legislative bulletin.

a mere bureaucratic exercise, stripping it of much of its potential to transform (Wismar et al. 2007; Esnaola et al. 2010).

The scope for HIA is loosely defined in most of the legislative texts (Table 15.2), except for the General Public Health Act, the Public Health Act of Andalusia, and the Public Health Bill in the Basque Country, where the use of HIA is being explicitly addressed as a tool to formulate healthy interventions in all sectors of the public administration. This aspect is related to the broader practical experiences observed in both regions (Table 15.1)

Health protection was already included under Spanish legislation regulating EIA. However, as in other European countries (Lock and McKee 2005), health considerations in this context have received only isolated attention, often leaving key issues unresolved or partially tackled. Andalusia has tried to redress this deficiency by extending the scope of mandatory HIA to public or private activities subject to EIA and to urban planning projects. The scope of its application in Andalusia could possibly be broadened in future legislative developments.

It has been argued that HIA cannot be implemented without suitable funding, especially when it is unclear who will bear the cost burden (Kearns and Pursell 2011). According to preliminary results reviewed by Kemm (2007), HIA's benefits far outweigh its costs. Wismar et al. (2007) reported that regular budget appropriations from national, regional, or local administrations to consistently sustain HIAs are still scarce in Europe, with some notable exceptions. Currently in Spain such budgets are non-existent and it remains to be seen what regulatory framework will emerge to strengthen these laws (Table 15.2) and provide the financial resources necessary to ensure HIA's effective implementation.

Another constraint to HIA institutionalization is the inadequate generation of information on health resources (data on population health and determinants), including intelligence for HIA in terms of concepts, guidelines, tools, evidence, and proper training (Lock and Mckee 2005; Wismar et al. 2007; Kearns and Pursell 2011). Currently, capacity building for HIA remains anecdotal in Spain (Table 15.1). The country's newly approved legal framework attempts to formally address this deficiency by promoting specific training in HIA for public health officers. On the other hand, establishing mandatory requirements for HIA could increase dependence on external sources of expertise, fostering the creation of a large number of consultancy firms. Smith et al. (2010) stated that this situation already exists at the policy-making level of the European Commission and noted that conflicts regarding consultants' impartiality and independence in the HIA process might also be present. Kemm (2007) suggested that a compromise should be reached between the need for a set of accredited skills among HIA practitioners and the need for a degree of flexibility that permits changes to be introduced into this continuously evolving field.

Establishing a lead agency to act as focal point for technical delivering is considered to be the fourth major category for triggering HIA institutionalization (Wismar et al. 2007; Kearns and Pursell 2011). Its establishment also ensures that the HIA and its recommendations will be reasonably impartial and independent. Spain's new regulatory framework takes this need into account and designates specific entities for conducting HIA. Catalonia, Aragon, and the Balearic Islands have assigned this task to their public health agencies while in Andalusia it will be assumed directly by the regional health department.

Opinion of key informants

Table 15.3 summarizes key messages extracted from an e-mail survey on factors identified as hurdles to the HIA institutionalization process in Spain. Seventeen people (81%) responded to the survey and messages were ranked according to those most frequently mentioned by participants. Factors were classified into two broad categories, one relating to the decision-making process and the other to the HIA practice. The greatest concerns highlighted in the former refer to how different policy sectors can address health values more systematically and effectively, the challenge of promoting a holistic approach to health, and the need to avoid the additional bureaucratization that occurred when EIA was made mandatory. The limited availability of economic resources due to the current crisis and the negative perception of HIA's cost burden are also cited as potential obstacles that could undermine HIA institutionalization in Spain (Table 15.3).

Overall concerns regarding inadequate resources and lack of qualified staff experienced in conducting HIA is extremely relevant and closely related to the reduced number of case studies found in Spain (Table 15.1). Respondents also deplore a history of unsatisfactory experiences involving inter-sectoral collaboration with health professionals, decision makers, and other public sector stakeholders.

Concluding remarks

Spain is attempting to make HIA legally binding in all public sector policies, in contrast with the situation in Europe, where this need is not being explicitly addressed. It remains to be seen whether sufficient political, financial, and technical resources can be marshalled to guarantee its successful institutionalization.

Table 15.3 Perceived hurdles to be surmounted to promote mandatory HIA institutionalization in Spain

Policy-making process in generating healthy public policies	Number*
Difficulties in promoting recognition of health considerations outside the health sector	7
The existing prevalent vision of health according to a biomedical model by health professionals, polity-makers, and citizens	4
Concern about reproducing past experiences involving other mandated assessment approaches (i.e. EIA), mired in an unproductive bureaucracy	4
The current economic and political crisis	2
Lack of leadership	2
Widespread negative perception of cost-benefits in conducting HIA, particularly outside the health sector	2
Little experience in incorporating public opinion into the policy-making process	1
HIA practice	
Lack of resources and qualified staff experienced in conducting HIA	11
Lack of experience in running inter-sectoral networks	6
Lack of an established standard method for conducting HIA	6
Difficulties in transferring public health research findings into an evidence-based analysis of the HIA process; gaps between science and the policy-making process	3
Disparities among regions in monitoring health and health determinants	1

*Frequency of response (number over 17 questionnaires)

Recommendations

Based on our experience, the following recommendations are suggested for achieving an extended HIA implementation in Spain:

◆ It is important that decision-makers would get involved at least at the HIA design stage, generating enough resources and an adequate organizational commitment for successful HIA development.

◆ Working partnerships amongst different stakeholders would be necessary for raising funding opportunities so HIA could be effectively implemented in the current context of economical crisis.

◆ More real inter-sectoral actions need to be promoted both at the political level and also at the technical level, avoiding an overall prominence of health values in comparison to other outcomes meriting policy.

- ◆ Public health experts should exert a stewardship role in facilitating that professionals from non-health sectors could implement HIA much more easily.
- ◆ Generation of HIA resources should be available in Spanish.
- ◆ Design of training programmes that would support capacity building should be encouraged.

Generic learning points
For public health practitioners and policy-makers

- ◆ Mandatory inclusion of HIA in a legislative public health framework is expected to incorporate HIA into the political-institutional agendas with a broad inter-sectoral approach.
- ◆ HIA institutionalization must be accompanied by financial resources.
- ◆ Past experience warns against unnecessary bureaucratization when implementing HIA and in favour of promoting effective multi-disciplinary networking, at both political and technical levels.

For educators and researchers

- ◆ Both quantitative and qualitative health impact methodologies within the HIA procedure are feasible approaches in conducting HIA.
- ◆ The implementation of extensive training programmes is identified as a crucial aspect in achieving a practical HIA institutionalization in Spain.

Acknowledgements

Part of this study was funded by the Regional Department of Economy, Science and Innovation of Andalusia, group CTS-177. The author is grateful to all key informants.

References

Aldasoro, E. (2009) *Screening process of regional policies in the Basque Country*. 10th International Conference of HIA. Rotterdam: Public Health Observatories. Available at <http://www.apho.org.uk/resource/item.aspx?RID=110331>. Accessed 8 February 2012.

Bacigalupe, A., Esnaola, S., Calderón, C., Zubazagoitia, J., and Alsadoro, E. (2010). Health impact assessment of an urban regeneration project: opportunities and challenges in the context of a Southern European city. *Journal of Epidemiology and Community Health* 64: 950–955.

Banken R. (2001) *Health impact assessment discussion papers: strategies for institutionalising HIA*. Brussels: WHO, European Centre for Health Policy.

Barroso, F. (2007) A private sector HIA initiative: a smoke-free workplace policy in Spain, in Wismar, M., Blau, J., Ernst, K., and Figueras, J. (eds), *The Effectiveness of Health Impact Assessment: Scope and Limitations of Supporting Decision-making in Europe*, pp 147–160. Copenhagen: WHO, European Observatory on Health Systems and Policies.

Boldo, E., Linares, C., Lumbreras, J. Borge, R., Narros, A., García-Pérez, J., Fernández-Navarro, P., Pérez-Gómez, B., Aragonés, N., Ramis, R., Pollán, M., Moreno, T., Karanasiou, A., and López-Abente, G. (2011) Health impact assessment of a reduction in ambient PM2.5 levels in Spain. *Environment International* 37 (2): 342–348.

Davenport, C., Mathers, J., and Parry, J. (2006) Use of health impact assessment in incorporating health considerations in decision making. *Journal of Epidemiology and Community Health* 60 196–201.

Esnaola, S., Bacigalupe, A., Sanz, E., Aldasoro, E., Calderón, C., Zuazagoitia, J., and Cambra, K. (2010) Health impact assessment: One way to introduce health in all policies. SESPAS Report 2010 (in Spanish). *Gaceta Sanitaria* 24 (1): 109–113.

Gómez, F. and Estibalez, J.J. (2011) Health impact assessment of the tunneling of the railroad in Vitoria-Gasteiz (Spain). XI International HIA Conference 'In times of crisis, healthier ways'.,14–15 April, Granada. Granada: Escuela Andaluza de Salud Pública.

González-Enríquez, J., Salvador-Llivina, T., López-Nicolás, A., Antón de las Heras, E., Musind, A., Fernández, E., García; M., Schiaffino, A., and Pérez-Escolano, I. (2002). The effects of implementing a smoking cessation intervention in Spain on morbidity, mortality and health care costs [in Spanish]. *Gaceta Sanitaria* 16: 308–317.

González, R., Martín-Olmedo, P., and Gijón, M.T. (2007) A prospective health impact assessment of the metro line in the city of Granada. [in Spanish] *Gaceta Sanitaria* 21 (2): 57.

Kearns, N. and Pursell, L. (2011) Time for a paradigm change? Tracing the institutionalisation of health impact assessment in the Republic of Ireland across health and environmental sectors. *Health Policy* 99: 91–96.

Kemm, J. (2007) What is HIA and why might be useful?, in Wismar, M., Blau, J., Ernst, K., and Figueras, J. (eds), *The Effectiveness of Health Impact Assessment: Scope and Limitations of Supporting Decision-making in Europe*. Copenhagen: WHO, European Observatory on Health Systems and Policies, pp. 3–13.

Künzli, N. and Pérez, L. (2007) Benefits in public health by reducing atmospheric air pollution in the metropolitan area of Barcelona, [in Spanish] Barcelona: CREAL. Available at <http://www.creal.cat/media/upload/arxius/assessorament/Informe_contaminacio_esp.pdf>. Accessed 8 February 2012.

Lock, K. and McKee, M. (2005) Health impact assessment: assessing opportunities and barriers to intersectoral health improvement in an expanded European Union. *Journal of Epidemiology and Community Health* 59: 356–360.

Mannheimer, L.N., Gulis, G., Letho J., and Östlin, P. (2007) Introducing health impact assessment: an analysis of political and administrative intersectoral working methods. *European Journal Public Health* 17 (5): 526–531.

Martín-Olmedo, P., Ballester, F., Nebot, M. Martínez-Rueda, T., Iñiguez, C., Daponte, A., Alonso-Fustel, E., Pascal, M., Declercq, C., and Medina, S. 2011) *Updated health impact assessment of urban air pollution in several Spanish cities.* Aphekom project. 23rd International ISEE conference, 13–16 September, Barcelona. Boston: International Society for Environmental Epidemiology.

Metcalfe, O. and Higgins, C. (2009) Healthy public policy—is health impact assessment the cornerstone? *Public Health* 123: 296–301.

Morteruel, M. and Díez, E. (2011) *Health impact assessment of buildings rehabilitation measures in a neighborhood of Barcelona.* XI International HIA Conference 'In times of crisis, healthier ways', 14–15 April, Granada. Granada: Escuela Andaluza de Salud Pública.

Oxman, A.D., Bjørndal, A., Becerra-Posada, F., Gibson, M., Block, M.A., Haines, A., Hamid, M., Odom, C.H., Lei, H., Levin, B., Lipsey, M.W., Littell, J.H., Mshinda, H., Ongolo-Zogo, P., Pang, T., Sewankambo, N., Songane, F., Soydan, H., Torgerson, C., Weisburd, D., Whitworth, J., and Wibulpolprasert, S. (2010). A framework for mandatory impact evaluation to ensure well informed public policy decisions. *Lancet* 375: 427–431.

Rojas-Rueda, D., de Nazelle, A., Marko, T., and Nieuwenhuijsen, M. (2011) The health risks and benefits of cycling in urban environments compared with car use: health impact assessment study. *British Medical Journal* 343: 1–8.

Rueda, J.R. (2005) *Guía para la evaluación del impacto en la salud y en el bienestar de proyectos, programas o políticas extrasanitarias.* Vitoria-Gasteiz: Investigación Comisionada, Gobierno Vasco.

Smith, K.E., Fooks, G., Collin, J., Weishaar, H., and Gilmore, A.B. (2010) Is the increasing policy use of impact assessment in Europe likely to undermine efforts to achieve healthy public policy? *Journal of Epidemiology and Community Health* 64: 478–487.

Ståhl, T., Wismar, M., Ollila, E., Lahtinen, E., and Leppo, K. (2006). *Health in All Policies Prospects and potentials.* Helsinki: Finnish Ministry of Social Affairs and Health. Available at <http://ec.europa.eu/health/archive/ph_information/documents/health_in_all_policies.pdf>. Accessed 8 February 2012.

Venegas, J., Artundo, C., Bolívar, J., López, L. and Ribadeneyra, A. 2011) *HIA of an urban regeneration project in Alcalá de Guadaíra: a pilot experience in Andalusia.* XI International HIA Conference 'In times of crisis, healthier ways', 14–15 April, Granada. Escuela Andaluza de Salud Pública, Granada

Wismar, M., Blau, J., Ernst, K., Elliott, E., Golby, A., van Herten, L., Lavin, T., Stricka, M., and Williams, G. (2007) Implementing and institutionalizing health impact assessment in Europe, in Wismar, M., Blau, J., Ernst, K., and Figueras, J. (eds), *The Effectiveness of Health Impact Assessment: Scope and Limitations of Supporting Decision-making in Europe.* Copenhagen: WHO, European Observatory on Health Systems and Policies, pp. 57–78.

Chapter 16

Integrating health into impact assessments in Scotland

Margaret Douglas, Susie Palmer,
and Martin Higgins

Introduction

Policy-makers may feel overwhelmed by the many impact assessments (IAs) that are required: environment, equality, human rights, business and so on. Health impact assessment (HIA) competes with other assessments and may be given lower priority because it is not required by legislation. As other issues being assessed are often health determinants, it can make sense to integrate health into other assessments rather than doing a separate HIA. This may reduce duplication of work and encourage 'champions' for different issues to work together on areas of common interest. However, health issues may be diluted if they form part of an assessment covering other issues; integrated assessments have been criticized for favouring business interests over public health (Smith et al. 2010).

This chapter presents our experience of integrating health into other assessment processes in Scotland. We will review the coverage of health in strategic environmental assessment (SEA) and the findings of a project that integrated assessment of health, equality, and human rights into a single process in Scottish Government and Scottish National Health Service (NHS) boards.

Background

Scotland is a country of approximately five million people. It forms part of the UK although has its own parliament, which is responsible for devolved matters, including health. NHS Boards are responsible for health service delivery and public health.

HIA has no statutory basis although the Scottish Health Impact Assessment Network has, since 2001, promoted and supported HIA in Scotland. The Scottish HIA Network is coordinated by NHS Health Scotland and is open to anyone working or planning to work on HIAs in Scotland (see <http://www.healthscotland.com/resources/networks/shian.aspx>).

There have been major HIAs conducted on regeneration programmes, planning proposals, wind farms, and the Commonwealth Games, but these have been ad hoc, in areas where there is commitment from policy-makers and public health professionals to conduct HIA and incorporate findings in plans and policies.

In Scotland, the Environmental Assessment (Scotland) Act 2005 modified the EU SEA Directive (2001/42/EC) so that SEA is required for all public sector policies plans and strategies.

UK equalities legislation requires public organizations to demonstrate that their policies promote equal opportunity and do not discriminate on the basis of selected 'protected characteristics'. The protected characteristics are age, disability, gender reassignment, marriage or civil partnership, pregnancy or maternity, race, religion or belief, sex, and sexual orientation. Equality impact assessment (EQIA) is used as a way to assess organizations' policies and functions to ensure they meet this legislation. EQIA does not consider wider determinants of health and is usually restricted to impacts relating to the protected characteristics, it will not consider differential impacts on people in poverty or other vulnerable groups.

In 2008 the Scottish Government published *Equally Well* (Scottish Government 2008), the report of the Ministerial inquiry into health inequalities. This included a recommendation to develop IIA 'with a strong focus on health inequalities'.

Health in strategic environmental assessment

The definition of health in Scottish SEA guidance is narrow. The SEA toolkit states 'the definition of health in the context of SEA should ... be considered in the context of the other issues outlined in Schedule 3(6) of the Act, thereby focusing on environmentally-related health issues such as significant health effects arising from the quality of air, water or soil' (Scottish Executive 2006). The Scottish HIA Network has argued that wider health issues should also be addressed in SEA. This has consistently been rejected by the government's SEA Gateway, which is concerned that widening SEA to include social and economic issues would dilute its role in raising environmental concerns.

The SEA guidance requires responsible authorities to submit reports on progress and findings of SEA, including an environmental report (ER) that details the issues considered and recommendations. We did a documentary review of 62 consecutive ERs submitted to the Gateway between November

2007 and October 2008 (Douglas et al. 2011). The review identified the health issues covered in the reports, the evidence used, and the extent to which it informed the recommendations.

We found that most of the policies assessed in the SEAs were from the sectors identified in the EU Directive. A minority scoped out health, but most included health as one of the issues to be considered in the assessment.

The SEAs identified criteria or objectives for each of the environmental issues and compared the policy against these objectives in a matrix. The SEAs considered a range of health issues—wider than just air, water, and soil quality—but this varied for SEAs of similar policies. In some cases the SEA assessors identified wider health issues but the Scottish Environmental Protection Agency (SEPA), the consultation authority for health, recommended that they be removed from the objectives. For example, SEPA recommended removing the objectives, 'Reduce and prevent crime and fear of crime' and 'Increase social inclusion'.

Many health objectives were fairly high level. For example, a common objective was 'To protect and enhance human health' without further specification of the relevant determinants. This suggests that the SEA assessors had limited understanding of the complex nature of health determinants—many policies could impact positively on some health determinants but negatively on others.

The use of evidence in SEA differed from usual HIA practice. The ERs presented a large number of other policies and a large volume of baseline data relating to each of the SEA issues. These were used to identify baseline 'environmental problems' and informed selection of SEA objectives. Very few presented any literature evidence. Apart from the consultation authorities, no stakeholders seemed to be consulted in identifying and assessing areas of impact. This may be because in SEA most consultation takes place following the preparation of the ER rather during the process of the assessment. Like HIA, the ERs used matrices but did not state what evidence was used to inform the judgements made in scoring how the policies would impact on each objective.

The most disappointing finding was that very few SEAs attempted to identify differential impacts. Several included an objective to 'reduce health inequalities' but did not outline the ways in which a policy might impact on different populations. Some SEAs of core paths plans (see <http://www.legislation.gov.uk/asp/2003/2/contents> for information) set objectives relating to 'access for people of different abilities', but did not state the particular population groups concerned. Only one SEA outlined how different populations might be affected in different ways by the policy. Notably, this was the only SEA that included a health impact scoping exercise.

More positively, we found evidence in the ERs that the SEA process had influenced the policies being assessed. For example, one reported that the SEA had influenced the decision to add a health aim to a local transport plan. This suggests that SEAs can influence change, and it is worthwhile trying to improve health coverage in SEA as a way to influence public policy.

The SEA guidance is now being reviewed. We will bring these findings to that review and continue to argue that health is wider than air, water, and soil quality.

Integrated impact assessment project

Policy-makers in Scottish Government are required to do EQIA for all policies and business and regulatory impact assessment (BRIA) for all new legislation. These use different processes but both require completion of templates that are published for public scrutiny. There is also pressure to implement assessment of impacts on human rights, carbon, and other issues as well as health.

The Equally Well recommendation for integrated impact assessment (IIA) recognized that an integrated approach could facilitate 'joined up' policy-making. However, established IAs varied in terms of processes and kinds of evidence used, and had a different values base from HIA, posing challenges in creating an integrated process.

We decided to combine HIA with EQIA and human rights IA. This integrated assessment was named health inequalities impact assessment (HIIA) (Palmer and Douglas 2011). There are obvious synergies between health, equality, and human rights—these are all about impacts on people. The Scottish Government Health Directorate had a commitment to review its EQIA process and increase the number and quality of EQIAs. The project was a way to achieve this objective. If the project was successful there would be an opportunity to influence the review and promote the new integrated approach.

The Scottish Government, NHS Health Scotland, and the Scottish Human Rights Commission formed a steering group. Two public health professionals with experience of IA (Margaret Douglas and Susie Palmer) led the project. Seven Scottish Government policies and three NHS Board policies were identified to pilot the approach. These were all health policies because the original mandate to develop this approach came from Scottish Government Health Directorates. However, they included policies at varying stages of development and of varying scope.

The HIIA process incorporated a scoping workshop for each policy in which a group of stakeholders used the checklist to identify the key affected populations and areas of impact of the policy. At the end of each workshop the facilitator summarized the key areas of impact and the group identified research questions and evidence sources to enable further examination of the impacts. A scribe took detailed notes and produced a workshop report.

The project team developed guidance and resources, including a scoping checklist (Table 16.1) to prompt identification of potentially affected populations and impacts on health determinants, equality, and human rights.

Following each workshop, the policy-maker completed the appraisal stage of the assessment. This involved gathering the evidence on the impacts identified during scoping, preparing an impact matrix, making recommendations, and

Table 16.1 Checklist for scoping workshops This checklist is intended to inform discussion to identify *potential* areas of impact. Further work will be needed to determine whether these apply and how significant they are.

1. Which population groups do you think could be affected by the policy?

How could these groups be affected differentially by the policy?

- Older people, people in the middle years, young people and children

- Women, men, and transgender people (include issues relating to pregnancy and maternity)

- Disabled people (includes physical disability, learning disability, sensory impairment, long-term medical conditions, mental health problems)

- Minority ethnic people (includes gypsy/travellers, non-English speakers)

- Refugees and asylum seekers

- People with different religions or beliefs

- Lesbian, gay, and bisexual people

- People who are unmarried, married, or in a civil partnership

- People in different socio-economic groups (including living in poverty/people of low income)

- People in different social classes

- Homeless people

- People involved in the criminal justice system

- People who have low literacy

- People in remote, rural, and/or island locations

- Carers

- Staff (including people with different work patterns, e.g. part/full-time, short-term, job share, seasonal)

- Other(s) (please specify)

(continued)

Table 16.1 (*Continued*)

2. What positive and negative impacts do you think there may be?

Which population groups could be affected by these impacts?

What impact will the proposal have on equality?

• Discrimination against groups of people

• Promoting equality of opportunity

• Tackling harassment

• Promoting positive attitudes

• Promoting good relations between different groups

• Community capacity building

What impact will the proposal have on lifestyles?

• Diet and nutrition

• Exercise and physical activity

• Substance use: tobacco, alcohol or drugs

• Sexual health

• Education and learning, or skills

What impact will the proposal have on the social environment?

• Social status

• Employment (paid or unpaid)

• Income

• Crime and fear of crime

• Family support and social networks

• Stress, resilience, and community assets

• Participation and inclusion

• Control

What impact will the proposal have on the physical environment?

• Living conditions

• Working conditions

• Pollution or climate change (waste, energy, resource use)

• Accidental injuries or public safety

• Transmission of infectious disease

How will the proposal impact on access to and quality of services?

• Health care

(*continued*)

Table 16.1 (*Continued*)

- Transport

- Social services

- Housing

- Education

- Culture and leisure

- Communicating information, consultation, and involvement.

3. Which human rights may be affected by the proposal?

Which population groups could be affected by these impacts?

Life (Article 2, ECHR)

Freedom from ill-treatment (Article 3, ECHR)

Liberty (Article 5, ECHR)

Fair hearing (Article 6, ECHR)

Private and family life (Article 8, ECHR)

Freedom of thought, conscience and religion (Article 9, ECHR)

Freedom of expression (Article 10, ECHR)

Freedom of assembly and association (Article 11, ECHR)

Marriage and founding a family (Article 12, ECHR)

Property (Article 1, Protocol 1, Article 1, Protocol 2, Article 2, Protocol 3, ECHR)

For details of issues considered for each Article see full checklist at <http://www.healthscotland.com/equalities/eqia/resources.aspx>

Adapted with permission from Douglas, M. and Palmer, S. (2011) Checklist for scoping workshops, Appendix 1 in Health Inequalities Impact Assessment An approach to fair and effective policy making, Guidance, tools and templates, Edinburgh: NHS Health Scotland. Available at <http://www.healthscotland.com/documents/5563.aspx>. Original 'Checklist for scoping workshops', Copyright © Margaret Douglas.

drafting the final HIIA report. None of the appraisals included quantification of health outcomes. They focused on assessing the likelihood and importance of impacts on health determinants because impacts on health occur through changes to determinants. Understanding these pathways is useful to inform changes to the policy that will enhance positive and mitigate adverse health consequences.

We undertook a process evaluation of the project to gather participants' experiences and views. The feedback was positive, especially regarding the scoping workshops. All participants reported that the process added value and 80% said the workshops had identified new issues, which was surprising as some of the policies were at a late stage of development or had already been implemented. Participants felt that involving a mix of stakeholders allowed more perspectives to be considered. They liked the structured workshop discussions and thought the scoping checklist allowed consideration of a significant number of potential health and equality impacts. Participants appreciated the focus on human rights impacts, but needed further support to determine whether they were significant. Most of the teams struggled to complete their HIIA report in time, partly because the pilot involved extra work that was not required for policy development or approval. Most participants said they felt confident to do another HIIA.

Overall, the approach was felt to be more creative and interactive than desktop assessments. It provided a wide perspective on the relevant impacts and informed policy development. Some improvements to the process were suggested, notably further prioritization of impacts before the appraisal stage. The guidance has now been amended to include this (Douglas and Palmer 2011). The facilitators have been asked to facilitate further scoping workshops on other policies. We are working to disseminate the use of this approach more widely in both Scottish Government and NHS Boards. Figure 16.1 shows the HIIA process as adopted following the pilot project. Full guidance materials are available at <http://www.healthscotland.com/equalities/eqia/resources.aspx>.

Ideas and practical solutions

Integrating health into other assessments is possible and helpful to policy-makers.

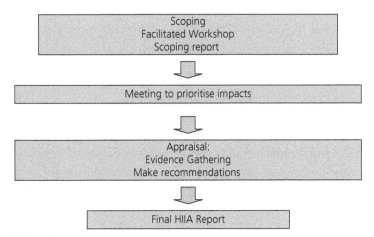

Fig. 16.1 HIIA process.

A workshop using a scoping checklist is a relatively quick yet structured way to gain different perspectives and identify relevant health issues. The integrated HIIA scoping checklist is shown in Table 16.1. A similar checklist can be used to identify relevant health issues in SEA.

This approach ensures that the evidence gathered is purposive, i.e. relevant to the identified impacts and useful to inform changes to the policy. It is helpful to have a follow-up meeting after a scoping workshop to prioritize the impacts and further evidence needed.

Conducting the scoping at an early stage in policy development can allow the IA to be built into the policy development process.

Conclusions

Policies in all sectors can impact on health, often in unintended and unanticipated ways. They may also impact differentially on different groups in the population. To influence policies to achieve better health outcomes, we must understand and assess their potential impacts on health. These case studies show that integrating health into other assessments has the potential to avoid duplication of work and can capitalize on the statutory requirement for some other assessments.

When developing an integrated assessment process, it is important to explore different perceptions of what impacts need to be considered and what forms of evidence should be used. The kinds of evidence used—even the meaning of the word 'evidence'—varies between assessment processes. Different assessments also involve stakeholders in different ways: in some, stakeholder views are taken as part of the evidence used to identify and explore impacts, in others consultation occurs after the assessment has been done. An early stage of the HIIA project was mapping the processes used for the assessment processes used in Scottish Government to identify similarities and differences.

It may be easier to integrate health into other assessments about impacts on people. The values underpinning different assessments may also vary. HIA is underpinned by the values of equity, democracy, sustainable development, and ethical use of evidence. EQIA is also underpinned by concern for equity and democracy. SEAs do not identify differential impacts and so do not reflect the equity value. These implicit differences in values may be one reason why it has been more difficult to integrate health into SEA than EQIA.

As in standalone HIA, scoping is crucial to ensure relevant impacts and affected populations are identified. A participatory workshop involving stakeholders is an effective and relatively quick way to do this, and can ensure that further evidence is gathered and used purposively to understand the impacts. In the HIIA project, participants reported that the scoping workshops were the most valuable part of the process. In the SEAs that were reviewed, the only SEA that identified differential impacts included an exercise using a similar scoping checklist with stakeholders. Adding this form of scoping to the SEA process routinely would be a good way to improve the coverage of health in SEA and also identify differential impacts.

These case studies have shown some of the benefits and pitfalls of integrating health into other assessments. If these approaches can be used more widely in a range of policy areas, it could help achieve better and more 'joined up' public policies and contribute to better health.

Generic learning points

For public health practitioners and policy-makers

- Integrating health into other assessments is feasible and can reduce duplication of work.
- Background work is needed to raise awareness of the links between health and other issues, and support the need to consider health impacts.
- Champions in other sectors can help break down institutional and cultural barriers.
- It is easier to integrate health issues into other assessments that are also about impacts on people.
- The scoping stage is essential to inform the issues considered.
- Scoping for health impacts should use a structured scoping process to identify potentially affected populations and determinants of health.
- A scoping workshop involving stakeholders using a checklist is an effective way to identify relevant impacts. Participants should include policy-makers and those who will be required to implement the policy. They should all be well informed about the policy ahead of the workshop.
- Scoping should take place early enough for the HIA to inform the relevant decisions but not before the proposal is sufficiently well developed to allow an assessment of its impacts.
- Following scoping, it is helpful to have a follow-up meeting to prioritize the impacts identified for further assessment.
- A small steering group should project manage the assessment and ensure it feeds into policy-making.

For educators and researchers

- HIAs should focus on impacts on health determinants.

- Scoping facilitators need sufficient knowledge and understanding of the policy and health determinants, equalities, and human rights in order to challenge and draw out particular views.

- It may be helpful to provide training and guidance on the issues considered in the checklist.

- Guidance to support appraisal of prioritized impacts could cover:

  - how to source, and quality assure, relevant evidence

  - how to deal with an absence of evidence.

- Monitoring and evaluation should consider separately:

  - the effectiveness of the IA in influencing changes to the proposal

  - the impacts of the proposal following implementation

References

Douglas, M.J., Carver, H., and Katikireddi, S.V. (2011) How well do strategic environmental assessments in Scotland consider human health? *Public Health* 125: 585–591.

Douglas, M. and Palmer, S. (2011) Health Inequalities Impact Assessment An approach to fair and effective policy making, Guidance, tools and templates, Edinburgh: NHS Health Scotland. Available at <http://www.healthscotland.com/documents/5563.aspx>.

Palmer, S and Douglas, M. (2011) The Health Inequalities Impact Assessment (HIIA) Project. A pilot of an Integrated Impact Assessment Policy Tool. Project Report. Edinburgh: NHS Health Scotland. Available at: <http://www.healthscotland.com/uploads/documents/15548-HIIA%20Pilot%20Project%20ReportFINAL%20(01042011).doc>.

Scottish Executive (2006) Strategic environmental assessment toolkit. Edinburgh: Scottish Executive. Available at: <http://www.scotland.gov.uk/Resource/Doc/148434/0039453.pdf>.

Scottish Government (2008) *Equally Well: Report of the Ministerial Task Force on Health Inequalities*. Edinburgh: Scottish Government. Available at: http://www.scotland.gov.uk/Resource/Doc/229649/0062206.pdf.

Smith, K.E., Fooks, G., Collin, J., Weishaar, H., and Gilmore, A.B. (2010) Is the increasing policy use of impact assessment in Europe likely to undermine efforts to achieve healthy public policy? *Journal of Epidemiology and Community Health* 64: 478–487.

Chapter 17

Health impact assessment in Colorado: a tool used to inform decision-making

Karen Roof

Introduction

Research and the practice of assessing health impacts within urban planning processes is gaining traction in the USA (Jackson et al. 2011). Public health can play a pivotal role in decision-making by considering impacts on physical and mental health, safety, social wellbeing, equity, and environmental sustainability of places. A comprehensive socio-ecological approach with interventions at various levels to collaboratively address public health issues on the part of decision-makers is both desirable and necessary. Yet, an understanding of how effective public health engagement can be within planning processes is limited. The emphasis of this case study is to evaluate how health impact assessment (HIA) can influence decision-making by determining the level of adoption of the HIA recommendations into the South Lincoln Redevelopment Master Plan, the amount of health language used in the master plan compared to other plans without an HIA, and other identified impacts and outcomes. This chapter contains a brief background on HIA in the USA, a description of the South Lincoln Homes HIA, an analysis of impacts from the South Lincoln Homes HIA, and lessons learned.

Dannenberg et al. (2008) examined 27 HIAs completed between 1999 and 2007 and by March 2012 there was a noticeable trend, with 152 either completed or in progress. The HIAs cut across policies, programmes, and plans that included after-school programmes, community transportation plans, and agricultural zoning (Health Impact Project 2012). Although the upward trend remains, the USA still lags behind the UK, Australia, and many other countries in the use and research of HIAs. This scenario is somewhat unexpected given that the USA enacted laws to regulate and assess environmental issues such as air and water quality but unfortunately does not adequately consider human health impacts (Jackson et al. 2011). The introduction of HIA to the USA is generally seen today as one of the principal ways to voluntarily incorporate public health into mainly non-health sectors (more details on the USA are in Chapter 8).

Colorado: HIA approach for improving housing redevelopment

In 2009 Mithūn, an architectural and planning firm and the selected master planner for the South Lincoln redevelopment, sub-contracted with EnviroHealth Consulting to conduct an HIA in Denver, Colorado. The City and County of Denver is the capital and the most populous city in the State of Colorado, with a population in 2010 of 600,158 (US Census Bureau 2010). In the South Lincoln neighbourhood, over half of the residents are Latino, and approximately 38% of residents and over half of the children live in poverty (Piton Foundation 2009). Located adjacent to an existing light rail station, this project aligns with the City of Denver's goal to expand the creation of compact, walkable communities centered around train systems (i.e. transit-oriented development). The project's vision is to transform South Lincoln into a green, healthy, desirable, and safe neighbourhood. The neighbourhood contains 270 public housing units and is proposed to become a mixed-income, mixed-use development with added public housing and new market value units that will triple the population (Schacher 2010). Gentrification is less of an issue with this redevelopment because residents who currently have public housing in the neighbourhood will have temporary housing close to the neighbourhood during the redevelopment and will continue to have public housing in South Lincoln when the construction is complete.

The purpose of the HIA was to assess current conditions, identify health issues and risks using evidence-based research and community data, and provide specific policy, programme, and built environment recommendations for the South Lincoln neighbourhood before completion of the master planning process. The collected data, other available documents, and information exchanged collaboratively with design team members were consolidated to form the HIA recommendations.

Data collection and community engagement

The HIA was conducted with the use of the Healthy Development Measurement Tool (HDMT) developed by the San Francisco Department of Public Health (2006). The HDMT is a comprehensive metric checklist with indicators used to consider the health needs in urban development plans and projects. In addition to the HDMT, evidence-based research, interviews, and focus groups with community members and organizations, feedback from an elected official, walkability and food audits, and data from two available surveys were utilized, along with agency data from several city departments (police, environmental health, planning, and others). Denver Housing Authority (DHA) funded, managed, and was the lead decision maker of the redevelopment. Additionally, the steering committee members included decision-makers from city council, multiple agencies, and community organizations, and nine of the approximately 26 members were community residents who regularly participated. Participatory strategies and activities were employed to build relationships between the residents and those serving them as well as to gather community input from and share information about the redevelopment.

The South Lincoln Homes HIA was a prospective activity that informed the master plan throughout the process and was completed before decisions were finalized in the master plan. As the HIA was being developed, drafts were sent to Mithūn and monthly presentations were conducted for the design team, steering committee, and the larger community. After the start of the HIA and master planning process in April 2009, an initial draft HIA was completed in June in order to provide the data that had been collected and issues identified. In September, EnviroHealth Consulting sent a complete draft to Mithūn for comments and the final version was made available to them in November 2009. The HIA was released in early 2010 with the master plan. This timing gave the planners within the City and Mithūn and other decision-makers the opportunity to learn about, review, and provide input into the HIA as it unfolded; although starting the HIA even a month earlier to provide more review and sharing opportunities would have been preferred.

Short-term outcomes

A number of positive outcomes occurred during the HIA process or immediately after completion. For example:

◆ Strong engagement by a city elected official after attending a presentation about the HIA at an early steering committee meeting led to policy change within the Denver Community Planning and Development (CPD) Department. CPD's requests for proposals for redevelopment projects include a requirement that public health considerations be addressed, although not necessarily through a formal HIA.

◆ During the early data collection period, the HIA assessor identified a free shuttle for community members to the closest hospital. Very few had been aware of the shuttle and since 65% of local residents lacked vehicles, this improved residents' access to health care.

◆ Other changes were less directly tied to the HIA process. At the same health presentation mentioned above, a portion of the discussion focused on reducing bike crashes and vehicle speeds by adding bike lanes on a wide, main community street. Adding bike lanes narrows the driving lane, which is an effective method of slowing vehicle traffic on the road. Approximately a month later, funding became available and was reallocated to construct bike lanes on the street; construction was completed in August 2010, one year later.

◆ Immediately on completion of the master plan and HIA, DHA paid to have the HDMT customized to improve the tool's applicability to Denver. Denver-specific changes and indicators, such as a consideration of water quantity, were added for the tool's continued use during the South Lincoln master plan implementation and for future housing projects.

Level of HIA influence on the master plan

The methodology used was an exploratory, retrospective case study using content and discourse analysis and in-depth document review mainly analysing the South Lincoln HIA and Master Plan processes and documents, along with other housing master plans. The evaluation focused on questions about whether and how well the HIA was effective at influencing the master plan. More specifically, it determined first, the level of health-supportive language in the master plan compared to three other housing master plans without an HIA completed, secondly, which of the HIA recommendations were adopted into the master plan by the decision makers, and last, potential factors that contributed to this. Other important information that was ascertained included the following:

◆ a determination of whether the HIA recommendations were partially or fully adopted

◆ whether the recommendations were considered likely or less likely to be incorporated into the master plan.

Content and discourse analysis of health language

Methodology

Determining the level of influence the HIA had on the South Lincoln Redevelopment Master Plan began with identifying the extent to which health-supportive language was incorporated in the plan. A content and discourse (to ensure context) analysis were conducted that compared the South Lincoln Redevelopment Master Plan, for which an HIA had been completed, with three additional housing master plans, for which no HIA had been completed. Besides South Lincoln, no other similar type of housing master plans was identified with a completed HIA. The other three housing master plans examined were the only ones identified through an online search for housing master plans; those with only diagrams, sketches, and very little text were not used in the comparison. The three plans were Yesler Terrace in Seattle, WA, Old Colony in Boston, MA, and Braddock East in Alexandria, VA. For each HIA, software such as ATLAS ti, a qualitative data analysis tool, was used to determine the frequency of health-related words such as 'health', 'bike', and 'physical activity' throughout each plan. Table 17.1 lists the results for the four housing master plans.

Findings

Results

From the South Lincoln Homes HIA, the words 'walking', 'physical activity', and 'HIA' appeared in the final draft of the master plan along with many other health-related words. The word 'health' appeared in the South Lincoln Redevelopment Master Plan a total of 26 times. This makes it the 39th most used word in the document (when removing common articles, prepositions, and words appearing in the title block). When combining words, 'health/healthy' appeared 42 times (two were taken out because 'health' was part of a title), making it the 19th most used term in the document. This places 'health/healthy' at the same high level use of words such as 'site', 'residents', and 'transportation', which would be expected to be used frequently in a master plan of a large redevelopment. The words 'health impact assessment' and 'HIA' were referenced 11 times in the South Lincoln Redevelopment Master Plan. This is important since the decision-makers of the master plan were not required to use the term HIA or even reference the document at all. It is encouraging how often the HIA was referenced, particularly considering how concisely the master plan was written and suggests that the HIA was considered worthwhile.

Among the four master plans, the South Lincoln Redevelopment Master Plan referenced health-related words most in all categories but two: Braddock East counts were highest for 'walk' and 'pedestrian', and Old Colony counts were highest for 'exercise'. South Lincoln, a 28-page document, had the most health-related words, with 225. Old Colony, a 115-page document, had a total of 137 health-related words. Braddock, with 88 pages, had 115 and Yesler, with 20 pages, had 34 health-related words. Based on these four master plans and

Table 17.1 Analysis of housing master plans

Master plans	South Lincoln	Yesler Terrace	Old Colony	Braddock East
Lead agency	Denver Housing Authority	Seattle Housing Authority	Boston Housing Authority	Alexandria Department of Plan and Zoning
Adopted	January 2010	May 2011	February 2011	October 2008
HIA conducted	Yes	No	No	No
Length	28 pages	20 pages	115 pages	88 pages
Health, healthy, healthier, healthiest	40	11	26	2
Bicycle, bike, biking, bicycling	23	2	9	9
Pedestrian, pedestrians, pedestrian-friendly	33	11	32	47
HIA	11	0	0	0
Safety, safer, safe	29	6	15	17
Walk, walking, walkways, walkable	22	2	9	37
Physical activity, exercise	5	0	8	1
Overweight, obese, obesity	2	0	0	0
LEED, energy star	12	0	7	2
Food, farmers market	48 Fresh food, healthy food, farmers market, food access, food audit, food production	2 Nutritious food, grow food	31 Food bank, food pantry, fast food, food co-op, food stamp	0
Total	225	34	137	115

Source: Data from South Lincoln Redevelopment Master Plan, January 2010, Denver, Colorado, USA, copyright © 2009 DHA—All Rights Reserved, available from <http://www.denverhousing. org/development/SouthLincoln/Pages/default.aspx>; Yesler Terrace Development Plan, May 2011, Seattle, Washington, USA, copyright © 2012 Seattle Housing Authority, available from <http://www. seattlehousing.org/redevelopment/pdf/DevPlanFinal-web.pdf>; The Old Colony Housing Development Master, February 2011, Boston, Massachusetts, USA, copyright ©, Boston Housing Authority, available from <http://www.boston.com/yourtown/news/Old%20Colony%20Master%20Plan.pdf>; Braddock East Master Plan, October 2008, Alexandria, Virginia, USA, copyright © 1995–2012 City of Alexandria, VA, available from <http://alexandriava.gov/uploadedFiles/planning/info/BEPlanFinal.pdf>.

the extent to which health-related language appears in them, the data suggests that how much health is a priority to the decision-makers, and whether an HIA was conducted on the project, are more contributing factors rather than, for example, the number of pages in the document.

Adoption of recommendations

Methodology

Assessing the adoption of the South Lincoln HIA recommendations into the final master plan required an in-depth review of the recommendations presented in the HIA and the master plan document. This process began by reviewing each of the recommendations in the HIA and determining whether the recommendation was feasible to be within the scope of the master plan, or less feasible to be within the master plan. All the recommendations were put into one of the two feasibility categories that are defined below. The following definitions constituted the adoption decision-making process that was also agreed on between the researchers and by the DHA project manager.

Feasible (more likely to likely) within master plan

♦ A recommendation that is within the purview of DHA and could be implemented without major assistance from outside agencies.

♦ Relates to a physical change to the built environment rather than a policy or programme (e.g. Recommendation 1.a from the HIA states 'incorporate attractive and safe streetscape amenities such as benches, game tables [and] decorative pedestrian lighting'. (EnviroHealth Consulting 2010)

♦ Referring to property on the redevelopment site.

Less feasible (less likely to not likely) within the master plan

♦ A recommendation that is outside the purview of DHA. An outside agency would have primary responsibility for implementation (e.g. recommendation 4c from the HIA regarding the promotion of the women, infants, and children programme; EnviroHealth Consulting 2010).

♦ Relates to a policy or programme (e.g. Recommendation 5n from the HIA suggests that the project collaborate with and support community policing programs and blight/graffiti elimination programs; EnviroHealth Consulting 2010).

♦ Referring to property that is outside the redevelopment site boundaries.

♦ Recommendations that are very detailed and better incorporated into the next detailed design phase.

Each of the recommendations was also rated by the DHA project manager to verify the results of the researchers. Table 17.2 shows the number of recommendations and their categorical break down. Once recommendations were classified as feasible or less feasible within the scope of the master plan, a determination was made about which of the recommendations were fully adopted and which were only partially or not adopted and were recorded in Table 17.2.

Findings

There are a total of 61 recommendations in the HIA that focused on built environment changes, policy, or programme considerations with the majority related to the built environment. The following are two examples of how it was determined that a recommendation was or was not feasible and whether it was fully or partially adopted.

1. The master plan incorporated part but not all of the recommendation. Recommendation 3b (feasible) is an example of this. It states in the HIA: 'Identify walking route(s) (1/2 and 1 mile) and collaborate with Santa Fe Artist and nearby students to develop signage markers to mark the routes and denote number of walking steps or mileage between certain destinations.' (EnviroHealth Consulting 2010) The plan identifies the ½ and 1 mile loops, but falls short of saying anything about signage. Therefore, it is only partially adopted.

2. The regulations do not allow it, yet the recommendation was fully adopted (less feasible). The recommendation states: 'Back-in angle parking provides safety benefits for lower speed roads such as 10th street promenade and 11th in front of the recreation center but currently city regulations do

Table 17.2 Recommendation adoption levels

Levels	Total number and percentage	Number adopted and percentage	Partially adopted	Fully adopted	Not adopted
Feasible	27 44%	27 100%	9 33%	18 67%	0
Less feasible	34 56%	10 29%	4 12%	6 18%	24 71%

not allow for this type of parking.' However, the master plan specifies more concisely that there will be back-in angle parking, as follows: 'On the north side of 11th Avenue between Osage and Mariposa Streets: back-in angled parking adjacent to Lincoln Park.' (EnviroHealth Consulting 2010)

Results

Twenty-seven (44%) of the recommendations were identified as feasible (Table 17.2). Of the 27 feasible recommendations, 100% were adopted. Eighteen (67%) were fully adopted into the master plan and 9 (33%) were partially adopted into the master plan. Also, of the 34 (56%) less feasible recommendations, 6 (18%) were considered fully adopted in the master plan and 4 (12%) were partially adopted, for a combination of 10 (29%) that were adopted and 24 (71%) that were not adopted at all.

Limitations

The author identified three limitations after going through this process. First, it was not clear whether the created classifications of the recommendations and the associated definitions for this evaluation were the most appropriate, such as 'feasible' or 'less feasible', since no other delineation had been established in prior research.

Secondly, this one HIA is not necessarily representative of all housing master plan HIAs and should not be generalized as such. Another example of a housing-related HIA is Trinity Plaza Housing Redevelopment, CA (San Francisco Department of Public Health 2003).

A third limitation is whether or not there is a correlation between the HIA recommendations and their adoption in the final master plan. For example, did the addition of a bike lane and other traffic-calming measures occur directly because of the South Lincoln HIA or because of recommendations from other disciplines? One way to determine direct or indirect impacts is through interviews with the decision-makers (currently underway) or identification of opportunistic impacts that can attempt to address whether the recommendations would have been incorporated into the plan without the HIA being conducted (Wismar et al. 2007).

Conclusions

The South Lincoln Homes HIA had demonstrable direct influences on the planning process and policies as well as indirect impacts. This suggests that HIA can play an important role in urban planning and improved decision-making, and be a catalyst for policy change. More specifically, the impacts can be an increase in health language, incorporation of health consideration in the request for proposal process, or adoption of recommendations that together support public health, safety, and wellbeing.

The South Lincoln case study is one of the few evaluations of HIA that has been published to date. The hope is that this study can make a contribution to the literature on HIA influences, utility, and effectiveness. The evaluation can also further increase the confidence of policy-makers and funders about some promising impacts and the value of HIA, but more evaluations are necessary to significantly enhance the field. This evaluation focused on whether decisions were influenced within the master plan but did not study if health awareness, knowledge, or attitudes were changed. This addition will provide an improved gauge of whether the HIA was effective. Additional evaluations also need to be studied and incorporated into a similar assessment model in order to ensure that results can be further verified and generalized. Such research will help advance the cause of improving community planning and continue to improve decision-making through the use of HIA.

Generic learning points

For public health practitioners and policy-makers

- Writing the recommendations clearly and concisely has been demonstrated to be important. Having specific recommendations makes it easier for planners and other decision-makers to adopt or implement them without a major rewrite. Many recommendations were incorporated fully yet were still more concisely written when put into the master plan.

- HIA practitioners need to consider the value of providing recommendations that are defined as 'less feasible'. It was surprising that 29% of those were adopted, suggesting support. Even if current regulations do not allow for the action, policy and regulatory change can still occur in the short term and/or long term, i.e. different decision-makers may be involved.

- Recommendations should be specific enough to give direction. For example, if a park, bike lane, or crosswalk is needed, provide pictures and/or exact locations so decision-makers are clear about the options. This can also assist with the evaluation process later.

- List recommended items separately so each one can be accepted, modified, or rejected otherwise they are less likely to be fully adopted.

- Prioritizing the recommendations is an important component and can be very useful when completed by the community and other stakeholders based on need, cost, time, etc. to better understand the needs of the community and provide more precise direction to decision-makers.

◆ Enable a cross-sector collaborative approach. The South Lincoln design team members included professionals from public health, building and landscape architecture, urban and transportation planning, real estate, community engagement, and social services. As literature supports, a blending of the responsibilities, tools, and perspectives of multiple sectors and the community can result in better health outcomes than when any one does it alone (Kochtitzky et al. 2006).

◆ HiAP should be considered as a model for an innovative, systems change approach by both governmental and non-governmental organizations. HiAP focuses on the co-benefits and win-win horizontal strategies, and explores and uses health as a linking factor for decision-makers whether in transportation, food, education, or environmental policies.

◆ The adoption of the HIA recommendations into a plan or policy does not guarantee its final implementation. Continued monitoring and evaluation must occur to determine whether the recommendations are later adopted during the detailed design phase or final implementation of a policy and plan.

For educators and researchers

◆ There is a growing need for more high school and college level courses to be offered regarding the connection between public health, land use and design, and HIA that supports inter-disciplinary learning. Educators need to incorporate joint programmes for students of schools of public health and planning and other departments or offer a concentration or certificate.

◆ Community engagement is a critical tenet of HIAs but can be very challenging, particularly among vulnerable populations. New tested tools, methods, activities/techniques, and policies are needed to more effectively engage with different communities at different HIA phases, mainly scoping, assessment, and recommendations.

Acknowledgements

The author would like to thank two graduate research assistants for their work on the evaluation: Chad Reischl (Urban and Regional Planning) and Beth Wyatt (Public Health) from the University of Colorado Denver.

References

Dannenberg, A., Bhatia, R., Cole, B., Heaton, S, Feldman, J., and Rutt, C. (2008) Use of health impact assessment in the US. 27 case studies, 1999–2007. *American Journal of Preventive Medicine* 34 (3): 241–256.

EnviroHealth Consulting (2010) *Health Impact Assessment: South Lincoln Homes.* Available at <http://www.healthimpactproject.org/hia/us/south-lincoln-homes>. Accessed 13 June 2012.

Health Impact Project (2012) *HIA in the United States.* Available at <http://www.health-impactproject.org/hia/us>. Accessed 21 May 2012.

Jackson, R., Bear, D., Bhatia, R., Cantor, S.B., Cave, B., Diez Roux, A.V., Dora, C., Fielding, J.E., Zivin, J.S.G., Levy, J.I., Quint, J.I., Raja, S., Schulz, A.J., and Wernham, A.A. (2011) *Improving Health in the United States: the Role of Health Impact Assessment.* Washington DC: Committee on Health Impact Assessment. Board on Environmental Studies and Toxicology, Division on Earth and Life Studies, National Research Council of the National Academies. Available at http://www.nap.edu/catalog.php?record_id=13229. Accessed 5 July 2012.

Kochtitzky, C., Frumkin, H., Rodriguez, R., Dannenberg, A., Rayman, J., Rose, K., Gillig, R., and Kanter, T. (2006) Urban Planning and Public Health at CDC. *Morbidity and Mortality Weekly Report* 55 (2): 34–38.

Schacher, T., Christensen, E., Benesi, J., and Antupit, S. (2010) *South Lincoln Redevelopment Master Plan Final Report.* Available at <http://www.den-verhousing.org/development/SouthLincoln/Documents/D.%20Master%20Plan-SoLi-FinalReport-JAN%202010%20-%20PART1.pdf>. Accessed 14 June 2012.

Piton Foundation (2009) US Census Bureau Data from 2000. Available at <http://www.piton.org/index.cfm?fuseaction=CommunityFacts.Search. Search Auraria-Lincoln Park>. Accessed 21 May 2009.

San Francisco Department of Public Health (2003) Trinity Plaza Housing Redevelopment. Available at <http://www.healthimpactproject.org/hia/us/trinity-pla-za-housing-redevelopment>. Accessed 21 May 2012.

San Francisco Department of Public Health (2006) The Healthy Development Measurement Tool. Available at <http://www.theHDMT.org>. Accessed 25 May 2009.

US Census Bureau, US Department of Commerce (2010) Interactive Population Map Available at <http://2010.census.gov/2010census/popmap/>. Accessed 13 April 2012.

Wismar, M., Blau, J., Ernst, K., and Figueras, J. (2007) *The Effectiveness of Health Impact Assessment: Scope and Limitations of Supporting Decision-Making in Europe.* Copenhagen: WHO Regional Office for Europe, pp 19–38.

Chapter 18

Lessons learned from health impact assessment experience around the world: where to next?

Monica O'Mullane

The purpose of this book has been to examine how the integration of health impact assessment (HIA) with policy processes can occur. The chapters have provided us with illustrative and insightful ways in which countries and regions have sought to align HIA with the relevant policy processes in a variety of creative ways. Taking the chapters together, the overview of HIA practice and research in countries across the world suggests several conclusions.

HIA practice and public policy

A number of key lessons and issues have been highlighted in the chapters of this book regarding the practice of HIA and its relationship with public policy, with the view for greater integration of HIA evidence and its process within the policy-making processes. This section will present the main themes arising from the book's chapters.

Engaging with all policy sectors

In terms of influencing policy and engaging with all policy sectors, the need for inter-sectoral action has been raised by various authors in this book based on experience in attempting to integrate HIA with the policy process. Indeed, inter-sectoral action is a pre-requisite for advancing the health in all policies (HiAP) agenda as well as promoting HIA as a means to achieve HiAP, as has been demonstrated in the Dutch experience (Chapter 12). It is important not to unduly raise expectations of what HIA can achieve when advancing it as a means of achieving HiAP. Along with the authors of the English experience (Chapter 7), it is sometimes more realistic to emphasize both strategic and methodological allied approaches that will health-proof policies and programmes, alongside HIA, in order to ensure that health considerations are included in policies. The context where HIA is being implemented is an important factor for integrating HIA with the policy processes—the institutional, legal, and political context. Champions for HIA within non-health sectors have been suggested as a means of dismantling any existing cultural and institutional barriers, as suggested by the authors of the Scottish experience (Chapter 16). In addition to this, champions for HIA in public health and health sectors are vital also, as public health is an identified leader for HIA, as are government ministries of health. Following on from this, consideration of a country's health system is important when considering the integration of HIA with policy processes and for its implementation. This was highlighted in Chapter 5, which compared the implementation of HIA in Denmark and Slovakia. The authors pointed out that HIA implementation must respect and acknowledge the public health system's traditions and culture. For example, some countries would implement HIA using a more top-down approach coming from the ministry with guidance for regional authorities, whereas other countries have a culture that is more responsive to a bottom-up approach, starting from the health authorities and associated agencies. Within the culture of some health systems there may be some resistance to undertake HIA since health authorities may believe health impacts are already considered within the framework of the system. This point was highlighted by the Australian experience in Chapter 9.

HIA practice

The practice of HIA, and how it can better enable integration with policy processes and recommendations for future change, is emphasized in all chapters of this book. The scope that HIA would extend to should be widened in countries where it continues to focus solely or mainly on physical environmental impacts, rather than being a more balanced operation focused on the wider determinants of health. Drawing from the African experience, as presented in chapter 14, it is important that national governments develop their own guidance and frameworks for HIA and do not only rely on international standards. This lesson is applicable across all countries and regions of the world. This would better integrate HIA practice into the daily business of national and local authorities. Scoping workshops for HIA or an impact assessment (IA) that includes health impacts should involve policy-makers, and a steering committee should be established that would manage the assessment and inform the policy-making process thereafter. This is a lesson learned from the Scottish experience when including health in integrated assessment. HIA recommendations should be specific and monitoring is at all times required as some recommendations' translation into policy may not occur, as was suggested in Chapter 17, drawing from the HIA evaluation in Colorado, USA. The authors of the HIA experience from Ireland (Chapter 4) concurred with this point, advocating that the more focused the recommendations are, the more likely they are to be integrated and used. As part of HIA practice, encouraging communities to be part of HIA can nurture civic empowerment, as noted in Chapter 11, based on the Thai experience. It is also important that those involved in HIA practice assign the same value for community knowledge, not only for scientific evidence.

Challenges in HIA practice

There are a number of challenges raised by contributors in their discussion of the practice of HIA. Indeed challenges are often of a structural (politico-administrative) and technical nature, as highlighted by the authors of Chapter 13. Challenges by and large refer to the requirement of individuals who have the capacity to conduct or participate in HIA, resources for the carrying out of HIA, data available for assessing health impacts, and appropriate time allocation to carry out the HIA. Health systems with a workforce capable of conducting an HIA are a necessary part of integrating HIA further into mainstream practice, as noted by the authors of Chapter 9 (Australia). Based on the African experience, the authors of Chapter 14 note that mandated capacity-building and resources for the conduct of HIA would ensure progressive development of HIA practice. Financial resources as a necessary part of comprehensive institutionalization for HIA in a country are vital for HIA implementation. However, in times of economic crisis and resource scarcity, creative ways and means are necessary to advance HIA, as described in this volume.

Translating from policy to practice

A key challenge to integrating HIA with the policy process is the utilization gap, as highlighted by the authors of Chapter 4 (Ireland). This gap refers to the lack of translation of policy recommendations to practice, which is an identifiable challenge for many involved in HIA practice around the world. In order to narrow and ultimately bridge this gap, it is important that HIA becomes 'business-as-usual' (Chapter 10) in national and local government. This can be done in a number of ways, such as fostering leadership from government ministries and local municipalities, developing a national HIA programme, incorporating HIA into national legislation and forming a ministerial HIA support unit. Indeed, garnering commitment in terms of political and administrative support from senior staff in health service agencies, and nationally from ministerial avenues, has been cited in this volume as being necessary for integration of HIA with public policy. The impact of this commitment can have a variety of effects, such as workforce capacity-building and training, resource allocation, and allotting the necessary infrastructure that HIA implementation requires. Accounting for both direct and indirect impacts on the policy-making processes is an important consideration also, as emphasized in Chapter 10 (New Zealand). Indirect impacts can include improved relationships with communities, strengthened democratic policy-making, and cultivated inter-sectoral collaboration. HIA, as a policy integration instrument and approach, can face difficulties in aligning and amending to public policy needs and requirements. The authors of Chapter 12 propose the solution of building consensus horizontally and vertically within administrative institutions and policy sectors to resolve conflicting interests. By building consensus, improved inter-sectoral collaboration can result, thus improving the acceptance and advancement of HIA.

HIA's place within parliamentary legislation

Many chapters referred to legislating for HIA. As rightly noted in Chapter 15, HIA becoming mandatory within national legislation is a controversial issue. On the one hand, legislating for HIA will safeguard it, by ensuring it will definitely be conducted in a country. On the other hand, HIA becoming mandatory has the potential of 'killing its spirit' (O'Mullane 2011) as it may be perceived as an administrative burden on the business of government management. Based on the Indian experience, the authors point out that capacity-building for the conduct and understanding of HIA must precede legislation that would require HIA practice. Such institutionalization would also be best accompanied by the instatement of an HIA support unit within a government ministry, as is the case in New Zealand, or the creation of an HIA Coordination Centre, as exists in Thailand. This support, especially within the framework of government ministries, could provide the necessary national leadership for developing HIA in a comprehensive way (Guliš et al. 2012). However, the occurrence of HIA legislation is the exception rather than the norm. Most countries do not legislatively require HIA and so, in the absence of legislation, inter-sectoral action must be made more manageable for the sectors involved in advancing HIA, as suggested by the authors of Chapter 8 (USA). Countries with no explicit HIA programme are required to act creatively when developing the HIA agenda, for instance by advancing it as an approach to address health equities within the health system, as was the Australian experience (Chapter 9).

Developing integrated assessment frameworks

Integrating health with other IAs is a popular subject for discussion and debate within public health and policy circles. At times, it all comes down to what is most practicable in each country context. In many countries, Environmental Impact Assessment (EIA) and Strategic Environmental Assessment (SEA) are already institutionalized and often this has paved the way for the inclusion of health impacts in EIA and for the development and institutionalization of HIA itself. The experience of Scotland in this matter is insightful, as described and discussed in Chapter 16. The authors presented experience in amalgamating health impacts and health inequalities impacts to form a health inequalities impact assessment (HIIA), the process of which was deemed more creative and interactive than a desktop assessment, as noted by the policy-makers involved in a project. The authors also emphasized the ease in integrating IAs that had a similar focus (such as health and equality). Integrated impact assessments (IIAs) can reduce duplication of work as long as the placement and importance of each of the foci of the IIA are not diluted and compromised. As highlighted by the authors of Chapter 13 (India), EIA guidance can have the potential to include the social determinants of health and health inequalities, also noting that developing health within the structure of EIA can lay a strong basis for advancing HIA in the future. Within spatial planning there is huge potential for improving public health by including HIA within the planning processes. It is also important to align HIA with local or national spatial planning priorities, making the path for further integration of HIA evidence into policy easier. Indeed, better joined-up policy-making can result from appropriately integrating IAs.

The role of research, education, and training

The role that research, education, and training play in implementing and developing HIA practice in countries across the world is vital for the future of HIA. This has been highlighted by the experiences shared in this volume. Such development would also ensure that health equity concerns and considerations are accounted for and often prioritized in research, education, and training in HIA. It was noted by the authors of Chapter 14 that what is also required is a greater awareness and understanding of health equity issues in research, education, and training.

Policy-makers' role in research, education, and training

It is vital to include policy-makers in research, education, and training circles because if we envisage policy-makers being involved in HIAs, their training and awareness of HIA and health impacts on the health determinants is an important aspect of HIA implementation. Creating HIA guidance without the input of policy-makers is in many ways absurd because if policy-makers are not aware of such guidance, or do not feel it is appropriate for their use, then it may gather dust on office shelves. Oftentimes in non-public-health circles, health is narrowly defined, as found by the authors of the inclusion of health impacts in national policy-making in England (Chapter 7). The conceptualization and definition of what health is, is a starting point for training and development with those formulating our policies. Indeed following on from this, it may often be the case that policy-makers are analysing health impacts without being explicitly aware of it, in which case fostering such awareness of the health impacts and their place in policy assessment is important.

Developing HIA capacity

The contributors to this volume repeatedly emphasize the importance of developing HIA capacity in order to ensure HIA implementation and thus paving the path for integration with public policy. Training and capacity-building are challenges that need to be addressed. Workforce capacity is vital in terms of boosting the knowledge and skills of the practitioners and professionals who would participate in an HIA. Indeed, comprehensive institutionalization of HIA, which would make integration with policy processes much smoother, would be much more difficult without the implementation of an extensive training programme. Capacity-building with a variety of stakeholders, from state- and non-state backgrounds, would strengthen HIA co-ownership, which is necessary for implementation. Capacity-building and training programmes must be adapted also by national countries and not simply replicated from other cultures, as highlighted by the authors of Chapters 14 and 15. Although international guidance on HIA would undoubtedly inform capacity-building across various countries, an appropriate adaptation needs to take place, with materials available in the national language. Raising competence in conducting HIA requires an active learning approach, as demonstrated by the Australian experience (Chapter 9). Capacity-building in HIA also requires training or re-training in skills such as programme and project management, and strengthening social skills such as negotiation and conflict management, as the experience of The Netherlands (Chapter 12) illustrates. A comprehensive national programme in HIA capacity-building can improve the translation of policy to practice.

Inter-disciplinary curriculum and course development

Related to the matter of capacity-building is the issue of creating and fostering curriculum and course development. Contributors emphasize that the future of HIA training and capacity-building relies largely on the development of inter-disciplinary training in educational institutions. Confining HIA training and education solely to the discipline of public health and health promotion is obsolete and not an appropriate perspective, given HIA's multi-disciplinary composition. Educators, and in particular those in positions of authority, should focus on including HIA education and training, as well as focusing on topics such as the social determinants of health and health equity. This needs to happen in both public health education and for those studying and training in the environmental health sciences, spatial planning, and the political and social sciences, amongst other disciplines. Lifelong learning and continuous training in HIA and associated approaches and instruments is a necessary ingredient for the successful implementation of HIA across countries.

Developing tools for HIA

Part of developing courses and curricula for HIA education and training is the need to put research energy into HIA methodological development. As many practitioners are aware, community engagement can often be a struggle to foster, as highlighted in the experience on HIA evaluation in Colorado, USA (Chapter 17). Development and research into new tools, techniques, and policies are needed in order to effectively and meaningfully engage community groups and advocates at all stages of the HIA process. This does not refer to the inclusion of community representatives in an HIA steering committee, whose participation is assumed to be the case, but more to engaging with the wider community in HIA. Continual development and testing of standardized screening, scoping, and risk-appraisal tools and checklists is a necessity in order to nurture the methodological framework for HIA, as emphasized by the authors of Chapter 16. In addition to this, training facilitators who would lead scoping workshops is also a vital consideration when developing methods. Without appropriate facilitation, by facilitators who have an in-depth knowledge of the policy in question and the role of the health determinants, scoping workshops may not achieve their full potential in terms of bringing stakeholders together and garnering appropriate knowledge and support.

Development of an inter-disciplinary research agenda

Following on from the need for inter-disciplinary education and training in HIA is the requirement for developing an inter-disciplinary research agenda, which would include relevant disciplines such as public health and health promotion, spatial planning, environmental sciences, and the political and social sciences. This can include the research and methodological development for HIA. This seems a logical sequence given HIA's multi-disciplinary nature. Fostering inter-disciplinary research which includes HIA would enhance effective considerations for health in spatial planning, as outlined by the authors of the Indian experience (Chapter 13). Given the fact that HIA is located at the intersection of different disciplinary cultures (for example spatial planning and public health), as emphasized in Chapter 6, the promotion of an inter-disciplinary research agenda at both national educational policy and institutional levels is vital for the development of HIA. This would also make the alignment of HIA evidence and its process with non-health-sector policies easier and more acceptable than is currently the case in some countries. Indeed, as well as promoting an inter-disciplinary research agenda, progressing national population health research agendas can also improve the receptivity of HIA, as highlighted by the authors of Chapter 8. Based on the African experience, the authors concluded that research was needed also for including health in IAs that are already institutionalized, which is a lesson applicable to many other country contexts. As stated already, improving the consideration of health impacts within instated IAs is a possible path as a precursor to HIA development or as a means for including health considerations. Part of research development is the need for the systematic evaluation of HIA as a research requirement. Evaluation of HIA can help strengthen and build its case, as highlighted by the authors of Chapters 10 and 17, as well as assessing the effectiveness of the relevant HIA or IA in influencing changes to the relevant policy or programme. This assessment should be followed by an estimation of the impact of the proposal in the post-implementation phase in order to track in as far as possible the impact of the conduct of the IA. This was suggested by the authors of Chapter 16.

Where to next? Informing the post-Gothenburg consensus on HIA

In many ways this volume is one reply to key experts and practitioners in the field, who called for those involved in the research and practice of HIA 'to come together to develop a post-Gothenburg international HIA consensus that moves the field forward' (Vohra et al. 2010: 1464). This book brings together a collection of experiences whose specific focus has been on the integration of HIA with the public policy processes. This first collection of such experience is a starting-point in this field, hopefully not the final book on the topic. Discussion and debate on the current practice of HIA and its role in shaping public policy and improving public health and wellbeing as collected in this volume may be one of the many strands of activity to inform the period of HIA practice we are currently witnessing, named by some experts as 'post-Gothenburg'. This refers to the seminal Gothenburg Consensus Paper (WHO 1999), as outlined in Chapter 2, which was produced by HIA practitioners and laid out the values and rationale of HIA at that time. However, as time has moved on so have the concept, composition, and purpose of HIA in countries across the world. This signifies the necessity for continued novel debate, discussion, and activity on the role of HIA.

Outlined in Box 18.1 are some areas of activity that we can, as a global community seeking to improve the consideration of health impacts in policies, engage with together. Of course this set of recommendations is not intended as an 'end-point' in the discussion of integrating HIA with public policy processes, but rather as a starting point for engaging all partners in the process in this endeavour.

Box 18.1 Recommendations for integrating HIA with public policy processes

International level

Given that inter-country sharing of experience can enhance the implementation of HIA, the continued and upcoming work of transnational and cross-sectoral partnerships should continue to flourish.

HIA, as a policy support approach, must continue to be promoted and used in the international arena.

Political commitments such as the Rio Political Declaration on Social Determinants of Health, which recommended the use of HIA as a means of enabling inter-sectoral work and improving public health, can be used when practitioners, policy-makers and all relevant professionals work together in developing HIA and the population health agenda.

National level

Government ministries should have the necessary infrastructure to assess policies and programmes for health impacts.

Training and education in HIA and associated approaches must take place at the national policy-making level.

Ministries of health, or another appropriate ministry, should establish and resource an internal HIA support unit/external HIA support agency that would take a leading position in implementing HIA throughout the country.

(Continued)

Box 18.1 (*Continued*)

High-level political and policy support

Pursuit and a fostering of an inter-disciplinary research agenda at the national educational and research level, which can support and develop HIA and tools for its conduct, is necessary.

Implementation of a resourced comprehensive training for HIA and associated approaches is essential to build capacity in assessing projects, programmes, and policies for health impacts.

All partners with an interest in the development of HIA must be involved in the development of research, educational, and training endeavours to promote inter-sectoral collaboration and enhance co-ownership for HIA.

Local level

Local government and health authority structures should have the necessary infrastructure for HIA implementation, whether in the presence or absence of legislation.

Capacity-building and training in HIA at local and regional levels

HIAs conducted at the local level must be supported either via an HIA support unit at a national level or locally through support structures in local government or health service institutions.

Summary

This chapter analyses some of the main themes and patterns that exist across the chapters of this book. These conclusions illustrate the variety of experiences and lessons regarding the relationship of HIA with the policy processes. It is hoped that these conclusions may act as lessons that will steer the future direction of integrating HIA with the policy processes. Recommendations for all practitioners, policy-makers, educators, researchers, students, and the wider community are presented, with a view to informing 'a post-Gothenburg international HIA consensus that moves the field forward', as described by key experts in the field (Vohra et al. 2010: 144). There are various challenges for HIA as policy integration tool, such as the meaningful engagement of communities who engage in the HIA process and the promotion of civic empowerment, engaging with all policy sectors, the translation of policy to practice, the challenges associated with HIA being legislated or not being legislated, the development of inter-disciplinary training and research for HIA, the relationship of HIA with other IAs, its use at local and national government level, the continued development of tools and methods, and the assessment of impacts on inequalities. However, despite the presence of these challenges, this book's collection of experience can inspire all those with an interest in integrating HIA with public policy to advance the field forward with gusto.

Bibliography

Guliš, G., Soeberg, M., Martuzzi, M., and Nowacki, J. (2012) *Strengthening the implementation of health impact assessment in Latvia*. Copenhagen: WHO Regional Office for Europe.

O'Mullane, M. (2011) Health Impact Assessment (HIA) and Institutionalisation: The Slovak Experience. Presentation at XI HIA International Conference, April 14–15, Granada.

Vohra, S., Cave, B., Viliani, F., Harris-Roxas, B., and Bhatia, R. (2010) New international consensus on health impact assessment. *The Lancet* 376: 1464.

WHO (1999) *Health Impact Assessment: Main Concepts and Suggested Approach* (Gothenburg Consensus Paper). Brussels: WHO.

WHO (2011) *Rio Political Declaration on Social Determinants of Health*. World Conference on Social Determinants of Health, 21 October 2011, Rio de Janeiro. Geneva: WHO.

Index

Note: page numbers in *italics* refer to figures and tables.